THAT BLACK
MEN MIGHT LIVE

THAT BLACK MEN MIGHT LIVE

MY FIGHT AGAINST PROSTATE CANCER

REVEREND CHARLES R. WILLIAMS
AND
VERNON A. WILLIAMS

HILTON PUBLISHING COMPANY
ROSCOE, IL

Copyright © 2003 by Reverend Charles R. Williams and Vernon A Williams
Published by Hilton Publishing Company, Inc.
PO Box 737, Roscoe, IL 61073
815-885-1070
www.hiltonpub.com

Notice: The information in this book is true and complete to the best of the authors' and publisher's knowledge. This book is intended only as an information reference and should not replace, countermand, or conflict with the advice given to readers by their physicians. The authors and publishers disclaim all liability in connection with the specific personal use of any and all information provided in this book.

Publisher's Cataloging-in-Publication:

Williams, Charles R., 1948-
     That black men might live : my fight against prostate
cancer / by Charles R. Williams and Vernon A. Williams
     p. cm.
     ISBN 0-9716067-3-0 (paper)
     ISBN 0-9716067-5-7   (hardcover)

     1. Williams, Charles R., 1948 --- Health. 2. Prostate
--Cancer--Patients--Indiana--Biography. 3. African
Americans--Indiana--Biography.   I. Williams, Vernon A.
II. Title

RC280.P7W53 2003   362.1'9699463'0092
                          QB103-200397

Printed and bound in the United States of America

Contents

CONTENTS

DEDICATION

To God Almighty, who inspired me to write this book

AND TO THE MEMORY OF MY FRIENDS:
Leo Madden, Corey Kelley and Sam Jones

ALSO TO:
My Stepbrother: Wade Anderson
My Uncles, all of whom are Prostate Cancer Survivors:
Major General Harry Brooks Jr. (Retired), James
Thomas Brooks, James Oscar Williams

MY CHILDREN:
Robert, Maisha, Ramone, Charles II, Andrea, Shakara

MY STEPDAUGHTERS:
Mache' and Nadia

AND TO
My mentor and former Chairman of the Board at
Indiana Black Expo, State Representative Bill Crawford,
the present Chairperson, Carolyn Mosby, and the
Indiana Black Expo Board of Directors who have all
been inspirational in my growth and development as a
leader. You have also shared in my professional struggles
as well as my personal challenges and have been instrumental in helping me to overcome them.

Acknowledgments

To my Mother Dorothy, and my Sister Kathy, who have been by my side throughout this battle with prostate cancer and who have been invaluable assets to me while writing this book. I say thank you an infinite number of times. Your love and compassion have been my strength. God has truly blessed me with your presence.

To my Aunt Betty, thank you for providing me with the knowledge of our family health history and giving me a greater insight into the benefits of alternative medicines. Your love, calls, and prayers have all brightened my life during some very dark days.

Thanks to my children, Robert, Maisha, Ramone, Charles II, Andrea, and Shakara, whose love and support has been uplifting. You are my major incentive in this fight.

A special thank you to my daughter Shakara, who is only eight years old, and who joined me in the creation of a public awareness campaign by producing her own commercial and participating in my billboard campaign to "Get Tested." And to my eldest son Robert, who disrupted his own life and traveled hundreds of miles to be with me, assisting me in any way he could to lighten the load of my day-to-day struggles. Son, I appreciate you.

To my very special lady, the love of my life, Valerie Parker, who counseled this first time author, and edited my first and final drafts. You have taught me the true meaning of unconditional love, intimacy without sex, and encouraged me to hope for the best, but to always believe in the victory, even though I may not see it. You were at my side even before the diagnosis, and have faithfully remained there throughout this journey. You have been my consciousness, recognizing my thoughts and feelings before I speak them. Your spirit and compassion motivate me. You have helped immensely throughout all of my challenges, helping me to face them strengthened, fortified, and encouraged. Thank you for embracing me with your love and sharing your light that shines so brightly and permeates my being. I love you.

Lynna Townsend, my Executive Assistant, and my best friend. You were with me each and every day, and have been a constant source of support and encouragement. You too are a source of my strength and someone I know I can count on to see me through.

Thanks to Attorney Joyce Rogers, Chief Operating Officer at Indiana Black Expo. You took the helm of my Presidency and carried on the great legacy of Indiana Black Expo, and were always there to support me and to keep me abreast of the day-to-day issues of the organization.

To Nicole, Filmore and Veronica, Indiana Black Expo staff members who support me above and beyond the call of duty. Thank you.

ACKNOWLEDGMENTS

A special thanks to my Pastor, Bishop T.G. Benjamin Jr., who has always been a brother, inspiration, and counselor to me. Thank you for your constant love and uplifting telephone calls and e-mails that always lift my spirit and provide encouragement. And to my Light of the World Christian Church family I thank you for your many prayers. They make a difference.

Thanks to Pastor Jeffrey Johnson and the Eastern Star Church family. Rev. Johnson, you have been a true Godsend, a brother and a friend. Your encouragement of spirit and love have been uplifting in my life for as long as I've known you. Your positive nature has been a contagious, major force in my fight to survive this disease. Thank you for always reminding me of the good things I have done to make life better for others.

To my Coca Cola Circle City Classic Family: Tony Mason, Tony McGee, Bill Mays, Joseph Slash, Gene Gardner, Attorney Larry Whitney, and George Pillow. My deepest appreciation for your prayers, support, thoughtfulness, telephone calls, and gifts of love.

To my many family and friends in Indianapolis and throughout the state of Indiana: Honorable Governor Frank O'Bannon, Honorable Mayor Bart Peterson, Guy Black, Dean Livingston and the Radio One family, Geno Shelton, Diane Penner, Bill Shrewsberry, Karen Wright, Anthony Calhoun, Attorney Richard & LaShawnia Benton, Jene' Cofer, Joyce Williams, Sherice Anderson, Elder Lionel Rush, Rev. and Mrs. Jenkins, Judy Walker, Addison and Nellie Simpson, Susan Gaither and family, Dr. Gene McFadden, Twyler and Tirre Jenkins, Mamie Ware, Linda Austin, Linda Cork, Al Hobbs (whose vision led to the title of this book) Bruce Bryant, Sue Gaither, Virgie Dobbs Scott Johnson, Rev. Jan Hall, Michele Johnson, Dr. Virginia

Caine, Health and Hospital Corporation, the Indiana State Board of Health, the Marion County Health Department, and the Indianapolis media, which gave me all the recognition I needed. All of your prayers, thoughts, and telephone calls have been appreciated.

To my many friends from around the country, Moses Brewer, Jim Thompson, Ivan Burwell, Jackie Smith, and Vanessa Williams. My deepest love for your tremendous spiritual support, telephone calls and prayers. Thank you from the bottom of my heart.

To my medical team of physicians and specialists. Thanks to Dr. Thomas Petrin, primary care physician, Dr. Andrew Moore, urologist, Dr. M.S. Murali, oncologist, Dr. Irene Minor, radiation oncologist, Dr. Keith Logie, oncologist, Linda Maynard, oncology nurse, and the staff at the Central Indiana Cancer Centers for a comprehensive treatment program and for teaching me about prostate cancer disease.

To Vernon Williams, my co-writer, whose dream it was to write a book. I appreciate you for your time, patience, guidance and skills. Your diligence to ensure the completion of my book has been a sustaining force. You have been a blessing to me. Thank you.

To my mentor and friend Rev. Jesse Jackson, whose love and support have been a constant inspiration in my life, Tommy Dortch, president of the national organization of 100 Black Men of America, and Kenny "Babyface" Edmonds, whose friendship and support have been an invaluable asset to me, and whose contribution to the writing of this book have been invaluable. I thank you all and want you to know that I truly appreciate you.

ACKNOWLEDGMENTS

But most importantly, to God Almighty, the one who created me, the one who will deliver me from the clenches of this dreadful disease. Thanks to the gentle urging of the spirit, I now no longer feel that I am a victim; I now know that I have been chosen. Chosen by God to go forth in the world among men and be the bearer of news that can sustain lives. I thank Him every day for the privilege and for His blessings. With regard to my illness and the creation of this book

"To God be the Glory."

MESSAGE TO THE READER

Prostate cancer probably touches every family in the United States at some level, and many other families around the world. And the word—cancer—almost always brings fear and a sense of hopelessness to many of those that it touches.

When I was diagnosed with prostate cancer, I endured all the shock and fear associated with the big "C." Because of my family history with this cancer, I know it can be a relentless killer. I wish I had researched my family's medical history before my diagnosis. Prior to that, I'd known my grandmother died of skin cancer; both my mother and sister, very recently, had breast cancer and survived, two of my mother's brothers, my father's brother and my stepbrother all survived prostate cancer. My cousin, my mother's brother's son, is also a cancer survivor. He had cancer of the thyroid. My aunt, my mother's sister, and her two daughters all have a condition called carcinoma insitu—which if untreated, will lead to the development of cancer. Unfortunately, it wasn't until after my diagnosis that I became fully aware of my family's prevalent history of cancer.

What I have discovered about prostate cancer and its treatment is somewhat frightening. It often leaves men feeling highly vulnerable and may lead those with prostate cancer to choose treatments that are not necessarily right for them. Like many forms of cancer, the medical community has different opinions about treatments, the subtleties of which are often not understood by lay people like me. Minorities, especially, may have trouble understanding conflicting opinions because they may not have access to medical experts, or may not be familiar with medical terms, or may not speak English as their primary language.

I worry about the average man who may not have the resources I am blessed to have. The cost of treatment is high. Access to computer technology for personal research is a luxury that everyone does not have at his or her disposal. Transportation may even pose a hardship for some. These resources are all necessary in the fight for survival. I thank God for providing them to me.

This book was not intended to exclude any man. The information in the book applies to all. But because we black American men have a higher incidence of prostate cancer and are more likely to die from this disease, the book focuses its message on the black community, specifically black men.

I can't overstate the importance of having family play a role in your efforts to conquer this disease. Prostate cancer can be debilitating both physically and emotionally. Your emotional stability will certainly impact your physical ability to cope with all of the setbacks, side effects, and results of your treatment. It is paramount that you not go it alone. Those who love you can help you research and investigate all of the available options, so that you can make the right treatment decisions for yourself. Their presence will help to cushion every blow, and be a constant reminder that you are not going through this journey alone, even though on the bad days you may feel that way.

This book was written during the period of my treatment. Corinthians 4:8,9 says that "We are troubled on every side, yet not distressed; we are perplexed, but not in despair; persecuted, but not forsaken; cast down, but not destroyed." This is the story of how God is carrying me through it all. The most important factor in this battle for your life is God. Know that he is almighty and ever present in your life and in every situation, good, bad or indifferent. As long as you have the faith, the substance of things hoped for, the evidence of things not seen, you can weather any storm. Adversity becomes a mere stepping-stone along the journey of your spiritual development. One thing I know for sure is that God has a way of working out his perfect will in your life. I know this because the Bible says that Jesus was perfected by the things he suffered. Hebrews 4:16 says "Let us therefore come boldly unto the throne of grace, that we may obtain mercy, and find grace to help in time of need." I am comforted by the spirit, and confident that even in this, God will see me through. He is the greatest gift of comfort that I can offer you. Men must become actively involved in the battle against prostate cancer. It is our lives and the quality of our lives, as well as those of generations to follow that are at risk.

Rev. Jesse Jackson, Tommy Dortch, and Kenny "Babyface" Edmonds provide invaluable information from a national perspective that confirms the need that all men get tested annually.

I sincerely hope that this book is of value to men newly diagnosed with prostate cancer as well as to men on the survival journey looking for renewed hope. I hope that it encourages all men and their families, and heightens their awareness of how imperative it is for them to join in the war against prostate cancer. And that war starts at home—with you, the reader.

FOREWORD

The American Cancer Society estimates there will be nearly 200,000 new prostate cancer cases diagnosed annually. It is the leading type of cancer among men by a margin of 2 to 1, compared to lung cancer, which is second on the list. Prostate cancer is also the second leading cause of cancer death among men, with upwards of 40,000 dying from this disease each year.

According to the American Cancer Society, "While the causes of prostate cancer are not yet completely understood, researchers have found several factors that are consistently associated with an increased risk of developing this disease. Among these are age, race, nationality, diet, and family history."

Black American men have the highest incidence of prostate cancer, and mortality rates associated with it in the world. The mortality rates for black American men more than doubles the mortality rate for white Americans, the group with the next highest level.

Prostate cancer seems to run in some families, suggesting an inherited or genetic factor. Having a father or brother with prostate cancer doubles a man's risk of developing this disease. According to the American Cancer Society, "The risk is even higher for men with several affected relatives, particularly if those relatives were young at the time of diagnosis."

Regardless of the known risk factors, prostate cancer knows no boundaries. It strikes men around the world, young and old, of all races and economic status. Ninety-two percent of men diagnosed with prostate cancer survive at least five years, and sixty-seven percent survive at least ten years. While these numbers may seem impressive, they don't begin to tell the complete story of the havoc that prostate cancer plays on many survivors' quality of life.

I was diagnosed with prostate cancer in June, 2002 at the age of 54. My cancer has spread to my bones, to the point that my physicians say I cannot be cured. But fortunately, I have another physician who has never lost a patient, and I am leaving the final decision up to Him, God Almighty.

When diagnosed, I was not interested in being just a "cancer survivor"—I sought a complete cure. I wanted all the cancer cells removed from my body and I wanted to maintain the quality of life to which I'd grown so accustomed. Men can be cured of this disease, and this was my ultimate goal.

The PSA (Prostate Specific Antigen) test now used to help detect prostate cancer was developed in 1984. This test gained widespread use for early detection around 1990. Since then, the prostate cancer death rate has declined. However, the medical community's position is that this drop has not conclusively proven to be a direct result of the administration of the PSA test itself. Most major scientific and medical organizations do not advocate mass screening or even routine screening for prostate cancer.

The American Cancer Society, The American Urological Association, and the National Comprehensive Cancer Network recommend that health care providers offer the PSA blood test and a digital rectal examination (DRE) yearly to most men beginning at the age of 50, and to younger men who are at high risk. On the other hand, the American College of Physicians, American Society of Internal Medicine, the U.S. Preventive Services Task Force, National Cancer Institute, Center for Disease Control and Prevention, American College of Preventative Medicine, do not advocate mass or routine screenings for prostate cancer.

I find it perplexing that the medical community is at odds on testing. The simple truth is that in most cases, if the prostate cancer is detected early, while still contained within the prostate gland, treatment options and the chance for a complete cure are much greater than when the cancer has spread. These are facts supported by evidence from the top prostate cancer research centers in the United States. Why then are there still medical organizations that do not support early, routine screening through PSA testing?

Prostate cancer can be a horrible disease. Even in long-term remission, there can be serious, debilitating side effects including impotency and incontinence. I believe the stigma associated with these side effects is the primary reason that this disease has, until very recently, remained in the closet.

Indiana Black Expo's Summer Celebration has the largest Minority Health Fair in the country. The Indiana State Board of Health sponsors the Health Fair. Every year we provide health care screenings for various diseases, including the PSA test for prostate cancer. Last year, after I went public with my illness, over 600 men received free PSA tests courtesy of organizations such as the Central Indiana Cancer Centers. Over ten percent of the men tested were at risk for prostate cancer.

God has inspired me to step forward and talk openly about my battle with prostate cancer. I have done television and radio commercials and billboard advertisements, courtesy of the Marion County Board of Health, that have inspired churches and community organizations, such as 100 Black Men and the Kappa Alpha Psi Fraternity to host prostate screening events.

Despite the conflicting views of the medical community about prostate cancer care and treatment, I hold this community in very high esteem. It has made tremendous strides in developing technologies and procedures to treat and cure prostate cancer.

Men have come a long way on the prostate cancer journey. I applaud Rev. Jesse Jackson's efforts to internationally address major health issues, and the national organization of 100 Black Men, for making prostate education and awareness a priority program throughout the country. With God's blessing, men will continue to make important strides. It is critical that we run the last mile of this journey. This "last mile" has to be a period of concerted activism. Women made breast cancer awareness and treatment a priority and they have done an excellent job. We must do the same for prostate cancer. Men must become catalysts to bring clarity to the detection and treatment of prostate cancer.

We should not be dismayed or dissuaded that our active involvement is necessary, but excited and relieved that there are truly good and proven medical treatment options available.

There is also our faith to sustain us. A faith based on the knowledge that God is with us in everything we do. He is the reason this book has been written and as we know, when God moves in a project, it is bound to work.

How do I know He is in this book? Because of the way it came together. After the public announcement of my diagnosis, I was invited to speak to a support group meeting for men suffering prostate cancer. It was held at St. Vincent Hospital in Indianapolis. Even though I had no idea what to expect, I was excited about going.

When I arrived, there was a room filled with forty men. All but two were black. I was pleasantly surprised to feel the camaraderie and sense of empathy everyone in the room seemed to share. I was on a panel of men who shared personal stories of coping with prostate cancer.

They asked that we each prepare a chronology of treatment and share it. As I sat listening to others, it was shocking to me that the other men had PSAs in the neighborhood of 10 or 12. Mine was more than ten times that. It shocked me into the realization of how serious my condition truly was.

I listened to all of these good men discuss their pain, their suffering, their hopes and fears. The one thing I didn't hear in any of the presentations was a reference to God or faith. When I spoke, I couldn't emphasize enough how God had blessed me throughout life and how I was letting the Lord order my steps throughout my fight with prostate cancer.

When the program ended, a lady at the back of the small meeting room offered books on the disease that were made available to members of the support group. This intrigued me since I had set out on a quest to gain as much knowledge as I could on prostate cancer. I shuffled through each of the books and the topics and reviewed the authors.

The young lady complimented my presentation. I thanked her. After completing my perusal of the literature, I nudged her and said in a jokingly serious manner, "I don't see anything here by or about black people." She responded in an apologetic tone, "There were no books available from the black perspective."

What she meant was that she wasn't aware of any books from that angle. Books written by black patients on the subject of prostate cancer were, definitely not easy to find. God planted a seed in my mind, at that moment, that there was a tremendous need for such a book, particularly when black men suffer so disproportionately from prostate cancer.

Suddenly I was obsessed with the notion. As soon as I got to my car, I grabbed the cell phone and called my writer friend Vernon Williams. He happened to be driving home at the time and agreed to meet me at a northwest Indianapolis restaurant to talk about this inspiration. When we talked, I recounted the experience with the support group and shared my inspiration with him. The fervor for the project was contagious.

I shared the book idea with Babyface. He enthusiastically referred me to Hilton Publishing Company owner Dr. Hilton M. Hudson II. God worked it all out, I thought to myself; Vernon would be the writer and Hilton Publishing Company the one who puts it all together for us. It all fell into place because God was in it from the start. It's amazing what this man-to-man support group inspired.

This book is the culmination of my legacy. With all that people may think I have accomplished in life (whether significant or otherwise), nothing compares to the potential impact of *That Black Men Might Live*. My prayer is that this book becomes the consummation of my legacy as it helps somebody—even one person—avoid prostate cancer or catch it early enough to do something about it; that this book prompts black men in particular to find out more about their family health histories and encourages them to focus on life's priorities.

INTRODUCTION

I don't even know what a good day is any more.

Saddled with the grim realization that I am in the most advanced stage of prostate cancer—it has already spread to my bones—I mostly experience bad days and "blessed" days.

The bad days are when none of the many medications or prayerful meditations help the pain. The blessed days are those during which there's at least enough relief, and strength within, to pray for the hurting to stop.

The worst of it all is thinking that there's a chance I could have prevented the suffering or at least lessened it. If I had only listened to the cries for help inside my own body, and the urging of my partner, I could have detected this dreaded disease earlier.

Instead, the prognosis from the medical team treating me is not encouraging. My kitchen countertop resembles that of a drug store. And my immune system has been weakened by chemotherapy treatment to the point where I consciously try to avoid large crowds. A person standing next to me who sneezes could put me at risk.

INTRODUCTION

I urinate a half dozen times or more every night; sleep is hard to come by. In response to the ultimate question, some of my doctors tell me that I may have only two years or less to live. It's enough to get the best man down.

But don't expect invitations to any "pity party" from me. I'm not having one. My future is inspired and I am brim full of anticipation. The buoyancy of my faith erases the pain like no prescription drug. On the bad days, the Lord carries me without my even being conscious of his presence.

It's amazing how the mind bolts with vigor even as the reluctant body winces—how the most abject suffering is eased by the presence of God.

The source of my optimism is simple. My predicament gives me the answer to the question of God's purpose for me in life. How many people ever get such a clear revelation and are able to know in their souls that it's true?

With all that I have accomplished after two decades of being blessed to preside over Indiana Black Expo, Inc.—one of the most successful African American organizations ever—it's clear that everything I've ever done in life has led me to this place.

Every thoughtful man and woman has occasionally pondered the reason for his or her existence. We all wonder what is the point of it all. Through good times and bad, even people of the most fortified faith question their past, present and future. People of good conscience want to be on the right path.

I am filled with a sense of God's purpose. Though every day the thought of dying haunts me, such thoughts pale in comparison to the realization of how my personal challenge is being used. My plight is nothing more than a weapon to fight a woeful problem—the way prostate cancer is ravaging our middle-aged and aging black male population.

I feel like a soldier marching as the Lord's drumbeat orders my steps.

Prostate cancer is a very treatable disease. Well-known individuals like famed pediatric surgeon Dr. Ben Carson, Harry Belafonte, Nation of Islam leader Louis Farrakhan, Andrew Young and Chicago Cubs manager Dusty Baker join millions of other brothers around the country—some of whom you may know personally—as living testaments to the effectiveness of treatment for those who are diagnosed early enough.

In the first stages of prostate cancer, a variety of treatments—including newly developed drugs and highly effective surgical procedures—are available. With some adjustments, survivors are usually able to resume their normal lifestyles after treatment.

I had my chance for that early diagnosis. Unlike many men who may suffer prostate cancer without any symptoms, my body was begging for help for almost two years before I finally decided to respond. Even after being told that indications suggested I had the disease, I foolishly tried to "play doctor" for months rather than follow the advice of doctors.

The result of that wait may be to suffer the ultimate consequence—death. Yet I no longer fear that. More inspired reflection reminds me that one of the great things about God is that He forgives. Though man holds us accountable in direct proportion to our blunders and, similarly, nature punishes any of its elements in conflict with its forces, our Lord is merciful and teaches redemption.

Thanks to God's grace, no matter what my timetable, my untiring faith and total submission to the Lord assure me that it's never too late. Romans 8:28 tells us, " . . . all things work together for good to those who love God, to those who are called to His purpose."

Even out of tragedy, God can be glorified.

In the beginning of my trying journey, I searched my soul and prayed relentlessly for purpose in my affliction. My joyously compelling duty was revealed in the lonely, sleepless darkness of night. God spoke to my spirit and said that through every means at my disposal, I am to tell my story.

Additionally, I believe my charge is to share the words of other brothers battling prostate cancer and, most importantly, admonish black men with every utterance I can muster not to do what I did.

Anyone considering my eulogy at this point is premature. I enjoy a special relationship with God and He tells me that my work is far from being completed. I haven't been stricken, I've been anointed. I haven't been cut down, I'm being lifted up.

God has positioned me to bare my soul, to join the chorus of those across the country who are pleading for African American men to be examined early for prostate cancer, to capture this killer in its tracks. My purpose is to convey—through knowledge gained out of the struggle of my experience—ways that this ravaging ailment can be prevented as well as treated.

It's a glorious feeling—like sunshine at midnight—to comprehend God's will so clearly even in the bleakest hour. No more do I waste time preoccupied with the menacing question, "Why me?" The answer is clear. Whatever happens with me now has to occur so that other black men might live.

So no matter how much I may flinch or grimace, don't think for a moment that I've given in to the prognosis of any medical team.

CHAPTER ONE

THERMOSTAT OR THERMOMETER

THE EVOLUTION OF LEADERSHIP

My battle with prostate cancer is consistent with my life before prostate cancer. Nothing ever came easily for me. And yet God gave me a lifetime of achieving what others told me that I couldn't.

Looking back on my youth, I would describe my earlier years as anything but normal. Then again, how do you define a normal childhood for a black man in America? It doesn't even matter. By whatever definition, the formative years for me were challenging.

My father, whose name is also Charles Williams, was divorced from my mother when I was just one year old. Except when he was around, family life was mostly forgettable. But I remember better days. Though we share the same first and last name, he is not senior and I am not junior. Even after he was no longer in the household, he was committed to being a good dad. My father and I maintain a close relationship.

All of my memories of interactions with my father are positive. He is a gentle and kind man, who loves his children and grandchildren very much. Even though he didn't drive, before my mother's relocation with my sister Kathy and me, my father would pick me up every weekend. I would stay with him at the home of his mother, Sadie O'Bannon. He and Grandma would both look after me and entertain me.

My father would take me to visit aunts, uncles, and cousins. I looked forward to spending time with dad because he was a very active person. When my father remarried and had more children, I would spend the weekends at his home with his family. My brother Kyle and sister Elaine and I became close to one another and we enjoyed hanging out.

My father was never a strict disciplinarian. He taught me that the word can be mightier than the sword and, without getting physical, taught me to respect and obey him. Even today we spend at least one day a week together. He goes with me to watch my son, Charlie, play football and basketball. He lavishes attention on his granddaughter Shakara, and goes with me to her activities, too. Dad visits with us all on Sunday.

I have the utmost admiration for my father. Those weekends together were the high point of my life until mom remarried and we moved away. I missed my father and wanted to go live with him. I guess my parents just couldn't agree on the terms because it never happened.

For most of my childhood, my mother and I lived with my maternal grandmother Nora Brooks. She virtually raised me. I have nothing but fond memories of her. Grandmother was a nurse who eventually opened and operated an Indianapolis nursing home. Despite her rigorous schedule, she always found time to impart wisdom and love to her children and grandchildren.

My grandfather, Harry Brooks Sr., couldn't have been more different. He was set in his old fashioned ways and didn't show much affection toward children. Grandfather died at fifty-eight from kidney failure, hardening of the arteries and diabetes. Grandmother died at the age of seventy-four from cancer.

My mother married three more times. None of the marriages worked. The cadre of stepfathers resulted in the instability of a family constantly on the move. There was little peace in the household during any of my mother's three tumultuous romances. I can't remember many times that we sat down for family dinner. And reduced to a dreadful blur are the hurtful recollections of my mother's bouts with domestic abuse.

I can barely remember all of their names, these men who trespassed on my youth. They came out of nowhere and in what seemed like an instant, were gone, except for the stepfather who moved us to Chicago from Indianapolis.

Each left behind scars of family disorientation with little hint for how a growing boy was to determine how "real men" should act—particularly how they should treat the women and children in their lives.

Disharmony in my mother's marriages may have planted the seed for the domestic discord that I would experience later in life. I witnessed my mother living very unhappily. As a result, in the relationships that I've had, if things got to a point where differences couldn't be easily resolved, they were over. I refused to live in misery.

Out of all the family adversity of my childhood came character building. In a sense, the lack of a consistent father figure forced me to assume the responsibility of determining my own manhood. It was the genesis of my evolution into leadership. When you can't turn to anyone else, you either languish in obscurity, accepting a sense of nothingness, or reject any notion of inferiority and search for ways to assert your self. In other words, you sink or swim, become a follower or assume the mantle of a leader. God chose for me the latter.

Born in Indianapolis, we moved to Abilene, Texas for a brief stay when I was ten-years-old. Then the family returned to Indianapolis. I have fond memories of days of what was then Indianapolis' only black high school, Crispus Attucks. The teachers were dedicated and the quality of learning was high. It was the school my mother and uncle had graduated from earlier. I wanted to graduate from Attucks, but my stepfather, who worked for the labor department, was transferred to Chicago, so we had to move again.

We lived in a modest south side neighborhood at 81st and Evans. The three-story apartment buildings were so close that you could reach out your bedroom window and touch the building next door.

I met Ernie Banks, the Chicago Cubs Hall of Famer, because his children's babysitter lived in our building. Red Saunders, musical director for the house band at the Regal Theater, lived on the first floor.

Our apartment was a half-mile from school. It was good exercise for me, because once I started school I got chased home almost every day. After a while, I made friends through playing football, forming a singing group, and just learning to win friends.

My grades were below average because I had no motivation to push myself. It was not that I was satisfied with mediocrity; it was just that I didn't feel overly challenged at Hirsch High School.

I had no clue where this maverick mindset was leading me, but I knew from the beginning that I didn't mind being different. I relished the ability to capture the attention of my friends and to charm teachers whenever I spoke.

The evolution of leadership during childhood was somewhat of a blessing and a burden. It wasn't long before I realized that if people actually responded to the things that I said and suggested, I needed to know what I was talking about. It was elementary. A misinformed person misleads, an individual with knowledge has the ability to lead well.

Of course, my perspectives on education changed as I matured. What I failed to grasp earlier was that well-honed learning skills, and an expansive base of general knowledge, facilitate any effort to grasp the big picture. I had mistakenly viewed education as an end before discovering that, in fact, it is a means to an end.

I developed an unquenchable thirst for useful information in every phase of life, but was even more convinced that for myself, the truth wouldn't be found in the classroom, on tests, or in textbooks.

As an adolescent, my obsession was sports and girls but my passion was singing. You couldn't tell me during that period just beyond puberty that the singing group I was in wouldn't eventually eclipse the legendary Temptin' Temptations. My dream was for our quintet to release one million selling hit after another. Along the way, I met David Ruffin backstage at the Regal, thanks to Red Saunders. Eight years later, Ruffin sang at my wedding reception. In him, as a star-struck teenager, I saw my future.

I could see myself on stage with one of those mustard-colored suits, coat open with a matching silk vest, skinny neck tie, patent leather shoes, and the obligatory "process" or "do" (a hairstyle popular in that era). The fellows and I would step to the beat, weave between each other, roll our arms and twist our heads, and gyrate our bodies to the feverish din of an auditorium rocked by the deafening screams of frenzied female fans.

In this fantasy, after a few encores, my singing group would dash from the rush of fans to a long black stretch limousine waiting just outside the backstage entrance. The chauffeur would have to wheel away cautiously to avoid the mob of adoring fans jogging alongside.

Invariably, in this vision, one of the finest of the young admirers would slip into the back seat and throw herself on me, without much resistance from me, until security managed to peel her away, stop the car and get her out. The life of a superstar is what, in my mind, awaited me.

So, while other boys at Hirsch High School in Chicago were wasting time with aspirations of becoming doctors, lawyers, teachers, preachers, scientists, businessmen, bankers, police, firemen, or astronauts, my reality carried me to one place: on stage, under the lights, before the crowd.

It didn't quite happen that way. But in a sense, the youthful vision was part of the evolution of leadership. Clearly, I wanted to interact with people. The dream persuaded me that I was comfortable on stage, in front of huge gatherings. The dream's association with the performing arts led me away from the "nine to five" career track. I couldn't imagine being confined to a single space for forty hours a week—just living for the weekend.

So these wistful dreams, cast off as ridiculous by more mature or less imaginative thinkers, had serious implications on my eventual pursuits. After all, a dream is the seed that needs to be planted for any future to grow. It was my youthful transformation as a visionary that would help me achieve most of my career goals.

The next aspect of my evolution to leadership occurred during my junior or senior year in high school when the Rev. Dr. Martin Luther King Jr. made his trip to Chicago to deal with the city's problems of fair housing and rampant discrimination.

I was always an emotional person. Whenever I would watch television during the 1960s, it intrigued and saddened me to see the brutal mistreatment of blacks in the South. Suddenly this larger-than-life African American icon whom I had only seen on TV was in town to speak at Soldier's Field. I was never so inspired.

Dr. King showed me that there was more than one kind of leader, and that all leaders essentially fall into one of two categories: thermostats or thermometers.

One kind of leader is a person whose primary goal is to tell the truth. His obligation is to research and gather facts and then give that information to his followers. The work of this learned individual is important because many black people can't get this information on their own. This kind of leader is a thermometer capable only of measuring what is.

The second kind of leader masters the first element and dares to take it to another level. This leader possesses the same wisdom, but something inside of him rejects the "go along to get along" in the black community.

These individuals are bold enough to challenge the system and suggest that people of color deserve everything that other citizens enjoy in this nation. They seek to set a new social and economic climate for change. These leaders are clearly the thermostats.

While Dr. King was definitely the quintessential thermostat—forging more change than perhaps any American of the twentieth century—he was always dealing with "thermometer" leaders trying to get him to ease up, sell out, accept conditions, or at the most, push for change as a slow, gradual process.

Of course this conflicts with the very nature of the "thermostat" leader who knows that gradualism is an unacceptable compromise when black people have been treated so badly and unfairly for so long. Once I fully understood the distinction between these two points of view, I knew that I couldn't settle for the status quo.

The black people in Chicago who were outspoken against the politics of oppression that ran rampant in urban America at the time were either limited in number or silent. Many of those outraged by City Hall were buffeted by "designated Negroes" who were allowed into the system. With a few dollar bills, hot dogs, and beer spread through the neighborhoods every four years, these people managed to keep many of the locals quiet.

The news media didn't seem to give much play to the African American groups and individuals in Chicago that were protesting the blatant racism and discrimination. Oppression of blacks there was as common as the elevated trains that rumbled the railways over the streets of the ghetto.

But then came Dr. King and his powerful entourage—which included Andrew Young, who later became the Mayor of Atlanta and a United Nations Ambassador, along with Rev. Jesse L.

Jackson, who twice ran for President of the United States and who founded Operation PUSH (People United to Save Humanity) and the Rainbow Coalition.

These men took a stand and commanded an audience. Dr. King faced off with the country's most prominent mayor, Richard J. Daley. Dr. King would not back down an inch from his convictions. He and his associates laid down a set of demands required to satisfy their grievances. In wonderment, I watched and listened as these eloquent black men stood up to perhaps the most powerful white man in America at the time.

Mayor Daley had the reputation of being the country's premier big city "boss." Presidential hopefuls knew that they had to come through Chicago and metaphorically kiss Daley's ring if they were to stand a chance of being elected. And yet this upstart southerner, Dr. King, had the unmitigated gall to challenge the practices of the Machine and challenge the legitimacy of claims by Chicago as "The City That Works."

Beyond his brazen courage, three things impressed me about Dr. King.

- First, he came to town and chose to stay in the poorer neighborhoods instead of the fancy hotels on Michigan Avenue. I saw humility.
- Second, he lived in Atlanta but was fighting for residents of Chicago as fervently as though he wanted to move his own family into that city's segregated neighborhoods. In that I saw selflessness.
- Third, reporters who relentlessly tried to twist his words only frustrated themselves. When they searched for contradictions in his strategy or philosophy, King's concise

and consistent dissertation thwarted their efforts. From that I saw principle.

My definition of leadership was refined further. I now defined it as the willingness to be out front and yet be humble, to put others before yourself and to speak in a clear voice on a foundation of integrity. Since he was also an ordained minister and pastor, Dr. King also taught me that a true foundation to lead is born out of commitment to God's purpose.

At that point, I made the decision that I would rather be the thermostat raising the heat on the establishment, than the thermometer content to tell it like it is with no vision of how it could or should be. I had no idea how God would guide my path, or how my natural inclination to serve would be fulfilled. I just knew that I wanted to be part of the movement and wanted to make a difference.

Up to this point, my life had epitomized the "bad boy" lifestyle. With all the quarreling at home between my mother and her husbands, I preferred the streets. Big city adolescence was an adventure. While I never got into anything that was life threatening or that landed me in jail, I got into my share of trouble.

My punishments were inconsequential. No sooner had my folks gotten past one incident with me, than I was into another. Maybe I was just restless. Maybe I was trying to rebel. Maybe the streets of Chicago were just too inviting.

I had no regard for curfews. My parents would insist that I make it home by 11 o'clock. In my mind, that was when the party started. I was strictly forbidden from having company when my parents weren't home. Not only did I defy that rule, but one of my friends stole our television during a visit. My stepfather went to his house and retrieved it, but I still got into serious trouble.

In any case, the prospects of my singing group reaching stardom faded as the individual troubles of different members of the group (and my own) started taking its toll. I just stayed in trouble. I can't exactly pinpoint the proverbial last straw, but eventually, my stepfather became fed up with my antics.

By today's standards of adolescent behavior, my mischief would be dismissed as negligible. My "old school" parents, however, had no intention of tolerating such insolence and disobedience. "Baby boomers" knew too well that when one of us got too far out of line, we had to be prepared to pay the price. There was no such thing as "time out" back in our days.

One day my stepfather angrily approached me wielding the leg of a chair. Lacing his speech with a few swear words, he told me he was two seconds away from going across my head with it. Only my mother's quick action stopped the situation from getting ugly.

I had finally run out of second chances. Not even my gift of gab would save me this time.

After calming down, my stepfather told me that since I couldn't seem to obey the rules of the house, it was no longer a place I could call home. My options were just as blunt. I was told that I could either go to a boy's school or enlist in the military.

It was a no-brainer for me.

My preference was the Marines because I liked the uniforms and the toughness of the Corps. I flunked the test for entry. I didn't care for the Air Force or the Army. The Navy was my second choice, though I hated the bell-bottom pants and those funny looking hats.

Because I had to get out the house I couldn't be too choosey. So the Navy was my choice. At least part of my decision was based on the assumption that I would be stationed close to home at the Great Lakes Naval Base, just outside of Chicago. Instead, I was shipped off to San Diego. From that west coast training base, I went to Vietnam.

Boot camp, sniper fire, mortar blasts, muddy foxholes, and a climate inundated with death and destruction are among the images I conjure up when I think about "the Nam." At the same time, I was blessed to be able to create another reality while I was there.

The three years in the military became my "boy to man" rite of passage. It brought my first personal brushes with racism. It taught me discipline in a way that I had never known. It was a crucial step in my evolution to leadership.

One of the greatest frustrations of African American soldiers fighting for the U.S. was that there was no music or entertainment available that reminded them of home. They saw a problem. I saw a solution.

I organized a Vietnam band competition for the troops featuring the best singing groups from the surrounding bases. I also performed. The show was a success. As a matter of fact, it was so successful that officials decided to take over the concept and bring in singing groups that featured soul music from Korea, Japan and the Philippines. They really weren't bad.

Having the idea stolen wasn't a disappointment. It was satisfying just to know that my entertainment concepts not only succeeded but kept growing. The experience was great because it provided my first glimpse into the process of event production. I would apply that savvy to my first few jobs involving promotions. In many ways, organizing and producing the concert in Vietnam was a precursor to responsibilities I would later assume with Indiana Black Expo.

This was the first time that I learned the value of turning a negative into a positive. My enlistment into the military was a result of needed discipline. My exit found me more mature, experienced and focused. To paraphrase one scripture, while someone else intended something for harm or "punishment," God meant it for good.

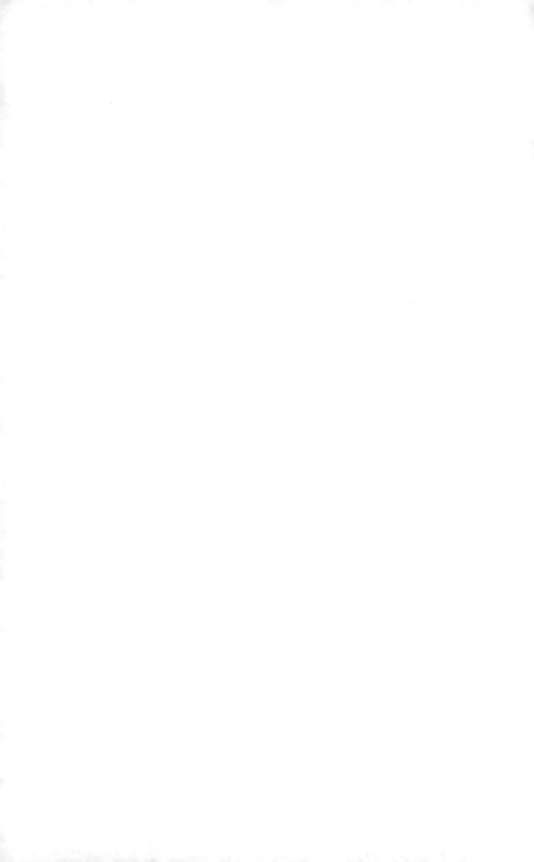

Chapter Two

DISCOVERING DESTINY

STEPPING UP TO THE CHALLENGE OF INDIANA BLACK EXPO

After being discharged from the Navy in 1968, I remained in Vietnam as a civilian employee for three more years. My first job out of the service was as purchasing agent for Alaska Barge and Transport, Inc.—the company that provided almost all the supplies to the troops.

There were no other minority employees for Alaska Barge and Transport, Inc. and the job paid well at an annual tax-free salary of $25,000. That was a considerable amount of money at the time. I was able to afford a full-time maid, a driver, and a part-time gardener.

One of the most memorable experiences of those three years came when I took a thirty-day leave to travel. I visited Copenhagen, Denmark, Stockholm, Sweden, Istanbul, Turkey, and Manila in the Philippines. Meeting so many different people with such diverse cultures broadened my perspective of the world and its people.

Upon returning to the states in 1971, I enrolled at Black Hawk College in Moline, Illinois. About nine months into my freshman year, I received a call informing me that the NAACP (National Association for the Advancement of Colored People) convention was going to be held in Indianapolis in 1973. They were in search of a local executive coordinator.

Word of my Vietnam band competition along with concerts and other successful events that I coordinated had begun to establish my reputation as a promising young promoter. The Indianapolis branch of the NAACP asked me to accept the job as executive coordinator for the convention. This was an exciting opportunity but I was also committed to getting my degree. Only after talking it over with one of my favorite professors, who encouraged me to complete my college education at a later time, did I accept the job.

I came back to Indianapolis in 1972, anticipating the wonderful experience that my new position would provide. What I discovered almost immediately were the finer points of my new job: There was no money for anything and there was no office space. I had to raise money for the convention expenses. I had never before produced any show on this scale. It was somewhat of a frightening challenge but not something that I would shy away from. I even had to raise money for my own salary!

The first thing I did was to organize a local committee of business stalwarts and leaders in the community. The next step was to call Motown and tell them we wanted to bring the Jackson Five to town. We telephoned their agent and booked the popular singing brothers. The concert was a sellout.

In addition to raising the first monies for the convention, we had the opportunity to get to know the Jackson family as we took Joe Jackson to a soul-food restaurant for barbecue and

Michael to a local mall to shop. It was a memorable event but, as they say, a taste of honey is worse than none at all. This experience only teased my sensibilities and increased my desire to stage more productions.

One of the most popular Broadway stage productions at the time was the black musical "Don't Bother Me . . . I Can't Cope." In an almost unheard of act, we convinced producers of the show to bring the original cast to the Circle Theater. It was a first for Indianapolis. Financially, we broke even. Communally, we prospered. We had sponsored the first black theater company to ever perform in this city.

In light of the success of these two productions, we began getting corporate contributions. By the time the NAACP convention convened, it was so impressively laid out and well executed that Roy Wilkins wanted to meet the young man who had orchestrated it. I was awed by his presence, but in our conversation I spent most of the time accepting compliments from Wilkins, who called the Indianapolis conclave the best the NAACP had seen.

The convention was a great achievement. It enabled me to cement corporate and civic relationships throughout the city and state. It proved to be the most significant bridge to later Expo successes. Unfortunately, I would be humbled in the interim when I found myself unpredictably out of work once the convention ended. It was a rude awakening and perhaps the most disappointing experience of my life. How could it be that no one wanted to employ such a promising young marketing and promotions prospect, who did so much with little for the NAACP?

Finally, a friend offered me a job with the state. The position required that I travel around the state and assess the needs of the poor. This may sound like unpleasant work but I met a lot of great people in the process and received an education about some of the conditions in which the less fortunate live. It would all contribute positively to developing the kind of empathy I'd require as a leader.

My next step was to work with the city. Indianapolis Mayor William Hudnut had an opening for a special assistant, and because others recommended me, my political life began. It also made me realize yet again that God was in all that I did; that there was an unavoidable destiny for me if I stayed the path of His purpose.

Out of that experience as special assistant came Indiana Black Expo.

Established in 1970 by black religious and civic leaders in Indianapolis and headed by the Rev. Andrew J. Brown Jr., Willard B. Ransom and James C. Cummings, the Indianapolis Black Expo (IBE) organization was patterned after a group that staged a similar event in Chicago under the leadership of the Rev. Jesse L. Jackson.

In the late 60s, Rev. Jesse L. Jackson created the first major black business and cultural expo in Chicago under the auspices of the Southern Christian Leadership Conference (SCLC) Operation: Breadbasket and eventually Operation: PUSH.

Many were skeptical about the plans for IBE, but Rev. Jackson was a believer and mentor to me from the beginning. In an interview, Rev. Jackson recounted the advent of Indiana Black Expo and assessed the future of the group in Indianapolis:

Working with Operation: Breadbasket, the economic division of SCLC, it occurred to me that when it came to black businesses many of our people didn't know who these businesses were because they couldn't afford to advertise, they didn't do much business with each other, and major corporations didn't see them as a market worth relating to.

After Dr. King was killed, we wanted to 'expose' our products. Then someone added the idea of exposing our talent, our culture and our children. So we devised a plan to come together once a year for this business festival. It was first called Operation: Breadbasket Expo before eventually becoming PUSH Expo.

Along with the business, we would bring in top entertainers from Motown, from New York, from Los Angeles, to showcase our culture. It became sort of the annual place to be for black Americans.

Many people tried to imitate the success of our event in various cities around the country. Charles Williams was the only one who captured the spirit of it, and institutionalized it, in Indianapolis. There had been others who tried to stage an Expo as a commercial idea. They have failed where Charles has succeeded.

Indianapolis has always been a special place. It is the place where Madame C. J. Walker lived. It is also the home of Oscar Robertson and Crispus Attucks High School. Indianapolis is a special place that may have been beneath some people's radar screen but I always knew it was a community with a considerable body of African American talent.

Expo is undoubtedly the piece of the puzzle of my life around which all the others fit. The organization has been my life. Through the grace of God and the tireless dedication of countless volunteers, staff and supporters, IBE has risen to become one of the preeminent African American organizations in the nation.

Sometimes out of the most unpromising circumstances will emerge the most marvelous manifestations of God's work. When you consider all the cities in the United States where you'd expect to find two of the largest ongoing African American events of all time, you might look toward L.A., Detroit, Atlanta, Washington D.C., Chicago, New Orleans—cities with significant black populations. Indianapolis would be at the bottom of most lists.

Yet the Indiana Black Expo Summer Celebration, staged every July in Indy, is the largest black gathering in the country with more than 300,000 attending from across the nation.

The list of those who have performed at, or attended, the Black Expo reads like an African American "Who's Who." Bill Cosby, Spike Lee, Muhammad Ali, Alex Haley, Vivica Fox, B.B. King, Stevie Wonder, Dick Gregory, Cicely Tyson, and Kenneth "Babyface" Edmonds are some of the best known. But these celebrities represent only a fraction of the star-studded list of participants in Expo's Summer Celebration over the past three decades.

The week-long celebration is highlighted annually by ecumenical services, a national youth summit, black business development seminars, an extensive job fair, prominent speakers, professional athletic competitions, concerts and cultural events, along with rows of exhibitors filling the huge Indiana Convention Center and the RCA Dome. Hotels are booked to capacity throughout a twenty-mile radius.

Money spent for hotels, entertainment, food, retail sales and transportation during the IBE Summer Celebration now exceeds $34 million each year.

A $150,000 grant from the Indianapolis–based Lilly Endowment allowed me to hire three staff people to work with me full time. IBE definitely needed to generate other sources of revenue to sustain and expand staff and operations. So while the summer celebration was our first significant success, a second idea began to crystallize.

It all started when, during my second year as president, I attended the Bayou Classic in New Orleans. The football game between Grambling and Southern drew more than 70,000 to the Superdome. I was always star struck by the legendary coach Eddie Robinson and amazed at how that massive event was so well organized and executed, not to mention how the astonishing bands brought the entire crowd to its feet.

Around that same time, Indianapolis was completing a similar domed stadium called the Hoosier Dome. I began praying for guidance on ways in which blacks could benefit from it.

My goal was to bring two black colleges to play in the facility, to emulate what had been so successful in New Orleans. To accomplish that, I went straight to the source. In a meeting with the president of Grambling and Coach Robinson, IBE invited that fabled black institution to participate in the inaugural Circle City Classic set for October, 1984.

Grambling agreed to play, but selecting an opponent wasn't as easy.

When I first approached the Lilly Endowment for seed money, the foundation was reluctant. It hired a consultant to do a feasibility study on the proposal; to determine if it had a chance of succeeding. The consultant concluded that the game wouldn't work unless Grambling agreed to play one of the area universities like Ball State or Indiana State. Unless we modified the original plan, the consultant insisted, we would be lucky to draw 15,000 people to the event.

Robinson disagreed vehemently and convinced me that Mississippi Valley would be a formidable, attractive first opponent. We went along with the coach's judgment and Lilly went along with ours'. Both decisions were right. For that kick-off Circle City Classic, more than 40,000 spectators—a sea of enthusiastic alumni, sports enthusiasts and folks just drawn to the hoopla—filled most of the Hoosier Dome.

Since then, the IBE/Coca-Cola Circle City Classic has consistently drawn between 50,000 to 60,000 spectators. Eventually, the Hoosier Dome became the home of the National Football League franchise Indianapolis Colts. Even after the arrival of the pros, the Classic was the first to successfully draw a capacity crowd to a football game in the stadium—which has since been renamed the RCA Dome.

The annual IBE/Coca-Cola Circle City Classic football game is now the second largest black sports event in the U.S. Following the mid-morning parade down the streets of Indianapolis, some 60,000 spectators fill the spacious downtown domed stadium for the game, which features a halftime show rivaling that of the movie "Drumline." After the game, about three times that number flood downtown Indianapolis streets, restaurants, tourist sites and nightclubs for the parties.

During the "Classic" weekend, the host city reaps another $24 million in revenue from participating locals and out of town guests.

The Summer Celebration and Circle City Classic are cornerstones of IBE, which boasts a national membership of more than

2,000. Less glamorous activities of the organization are just as significant, including the annual IBE scholarship program that has awarded more than a million dollars for tuition and other college expenses to African American scholars throughout the state.

The "Feed The Hungry" initiative is a less ballyhooed, but just as critical, program that addresses the needs of less fortunate Indianapolis residents. Ongoing components of the IBE youth initiative include the Youth Video Institute, which produces a teen talk program entitled "360 Degrees" that airs on local television as well as a countywide student stock market club, sponsored in conjunction with the *Indianapolis Star*, that teaches public school students how to invest and manage their money. With its myriad programs, easily the most gratifying activity of IBE has always been the public health fair held during the Summer Celebration.

Each year thousands of people participate in screenings for HIV/AIDS, STDs, sickle cell disease, cholesterol, diabetes, glaucoma, breast cancer, asthma, hypertension, hearing disorders, dental problems and prostate cancer—tests that would easily cost participants thousands of dollars. During the summer extravaganza, these examinations are provided free.

Ironically, I walk through the health fair every year and every year I publicly express gratitude for the hard work of the medical volunteers. Through the years, I always took time to meet and greet, praising the wisdom of those who patiently waited in long lines to be screened. And I marveled at the way in which the program's services expanded each year.

I did everything but the one thing I should've done—take the tests myself. I would step briskly through the crowd—too fast to stop long enough to get my own check-up. No time. Just, no time. Excuses. Excuses. Excuses. It makes you wonder if some people would find a way out of being tested even if doctors backed a mobile PSA examination unit up to their door and brought all the equipment into their living room.

We do what we really want to do—within our means. The rest we get to whenever we "can make the time" or "secure the funds," or we wind up putting it off altogether.

News of my illness broke about two or three weeks before the 2002 summer celebration's health fair. Kappa Alpha Psi Fraternity had already taken the lead in advocating that black men take PSA tests. Frat brothers manned the health fair booth where information and registration forms were distributed.

The effort was an overwhelming success. A record 600 men were given a PSA test during the summer celebration. Thirty tested positive! Early discovery of prostate cancer enabled these men to seek out, and get, prompt medical attention. Such prompt attention can mean the difference between life and death, and that's the kind of thing that happens every year during the event. The health fair is the quintessential 'people helping people' activity.

The annual health fair is an inspired collaboration between the Indiana State Board of Health, the Marion County Health Commission, City of Indianapolis health officials and local health care providers. It exemplifies the many partnerships between business, industry, government and other organizations that Indiana Black Expo has forged since its inception. The strength of IBE is its ability to combine resources for a common good. Again, it was a matter of God making all the pieces of the puzzle fit together.

Sometimes, though, a fragment of the puzzle that doesn't seem to fit turns out to be the centerpiece. Who could predict that an under achiever in grade school, who then became an adolescent malcontent a few seconds from being carted off to boy's reformatory school, would now be a galvanizing force for a powerful black health initiative?

But though folks on the outside looking in might have considered me unlikely in that role, I always knew that God had a special purpose for me. The Master knew that everything I went through, good and bad, was leading to Expo.

The road to prominence wasn't without its potholes and bumps for IBE, which was originally called Indianapolis Black Expo. Three years later, the name was changed to Indiana Black Expo and the focus—to serve the needs of more blacks around the state—was intensified.

IBE chapters were formed in African American communities in several of the major Indiana cities. Dedicated, hard-working volunteers provided a support network for IBE and were the source of early successes. But as the concept grew, so did its needs. Expo outgrew its ability to function effectively as an all-volunteer organization.

My involvement with IBE started in 1978. In 1980, I was elected Chairman of the Board. At the time, IBE was $106,000 in the red. With a coalition of concerned individuals, I was able to devise a plan that effectively retired the debt. I did this by getting creditors either to extend the time allotted for payment, forgive debts altogether, or allow Expo to barter and give them a trade off for the amount owed.

In 1983, I was asked to become the first full–time salaried president of Indiana Black Expo. The timing of the offer was ironic because Rev. Jackson had just visited Indianapolis and offered me a job as vice-president of PUSH. It was an intriguing offer worthy of serious consideration. After all, it would have provided an opportunity to work with one of my true mentors.

At the same time, I was employed as special assistant to Indianapolis Mayor William Hudnut. Was the position with IBE worth the risk of my seemingly more secure job status with the city? Despite some reservations, after earnest prayer and consultations with people I trusted, I decided to accept the IBE presidency and the challenge that came with it. It was a decision I never regretted.

January 1983 marked the beginning of a new era with the organization. It was the genesis of new prospects.

With the success of IBE, the staff has grown from the original three to twenty two and counting. Where we started out more than $100,000 in debt, the organization's 2003 operating budget exceeded $4.2 million. IBE battled through the financial challenges of the 1980s and worked with a sizeable grant from Lilly to put together a five-year strategic plan to better organize Expo's structure, operations and management. The plan was effective. The organization had never operated more smoothly.

One lesson learned in leadership is that along with the accolades and glory, a person has to be willing to accept the cheap shots and accusations. Part of what makes me strong in the face of being diagnosed with prostate cancer is the variety of adverse experiences I've had between the IBE successes. If nothing else, I learned how to take a punch and come back fighting.

The one thing that none of my adversaries can claim is that I dodged controversy or tried to evade the issues. No matter how unjust or unwarranted the claim, IBE stepped forward to field criticism. Even when it became personal I always knew that whenever you strive to serve the Lord, you anger Satan. Still, isn't it true that no weapon formed against God's people shall prosper and that the suffering of the righteous is redemptive?

There have been moments when Expo was down, but never out. Even when my heart was heavy, my spirit was never broken.

I think back on the leaders I've admired, respected, and initially patterned my ideologies upon in the early years of IBE. How many times did Rev. Dr. King and Rev. Jackson stand alone in their visionary beliefs? Yet, to be an effective leader one must be able to reach one's followers; one voice must give way to many. Rev. Jackson expressed this in reference to the condition in which I now find myself. He explained it like this:

African Americans listen mostly to disc jockeys on the radio and ministers in the pulpit. Those who have the microphones have the most responsibility to educate others regarding prostate cancer. Entertainers, popular athletes and other high profile individuals should get involved. Those who have the light must be willing to shine theirs' in dark places.

Rev. Jackson has always been willing to carry the torch. I'll never forget the time that he was coming to Indianapolis and wanted to promote HIV/AIDS awareness. He believed then, as he does now, that we have to call on those persons in our community who have voices if we want important messages to spread.

Yet Jesse and I learned that getting the church leaders to step up to the plate on touchy health issues isn't easy. Many people were afraid to take the HIV test because they feared a breach of confidentiality. We wanted to eliminate the fear factor by having a dignified and respected institution lead the charge for testing and treatment.

As ecumenical speaker for the Summer Celebration, Rev. Jackson called to see if we could convene an impressive gathering of ministers for the press conference who would be willing to urge their parishioners to be tested for HIV and AIDS. The idea was to get ministers to lead the way by volunteering for the tests; to teach by example how important it is for people to be aware of, as well as to be tested for, HIV and AIDS.

My executive assistant called around to ministers friendly to Expo and the heads of several ministerial alliances. They were asked to attend the brief press conference the day before the ecumenical service at Light of the World Christian Church to promote the Summer Celebration, ecumenical service and, most importantly, HIV/AIDS awareness.

Running late, I called to the office to check on responses to the invitation. I was stunned to find out that not a single minister had agreed to participate. Even on short notice, these leading clergymen have been known to accommodate individuals of the stature of Rev. Jackson. I couldn't believe it.

When I got to the church, no one was there but Jesse and me. The media assembled and asked questions as planned. However, the united front against HIV/AIDS couldn't be staged for the cameras. It was such a disappointment for me. I would never have imagined, and you couldn't have convinced me, that not one local minister would show up to support the cause.

When all the news reporters cleared the room, we sat down. I told Rev. Jackson that I had no explanation for the "no shows." He did. He reminded me that AIDS was still a very touchy, controversial subject because so many people were unfamiliar with the facts. Many ministers feel ill equipped to broach subjects that they know little about.

Rev. Jackson came up with an alternate plan.

On the night of the ecumenical service, he called all ministers and elected officials to the altar. They unsuspectingly made their way to the front of the crowd of some 2,000 gathered for the event. Rev. Jackson surprised the respondents by asking them to lead the way and take the HIV/AIDS tests that night. We had already arranged for the health department to set up in the lobby. Mayor Bart Peterson led the way.

When people saw the mayor, ministers and public officials taking the swab and volunteering to be tested, it motivated hundreds to follow. We don't know how many people took the test, but most did. It was almost more than the health department staff could handle.

The sight of so many black people getting the message and responding in such a positive spirit was breathtaking. The moving scene that night reminded me of how instrumental IBE can be when it comes to raising awareness about health concerns.

Even when people get past the mental blocks about health testing, making the time to do it is still a concern. Rev. Jackson uses the analogy of Earvin "Magic" Johnson's situation to make a parallel. The "Country Preacher" points out:

There is not nearly enough commitment among black men to get cancer tests or HIV/AIDS tests. Early detection is the best shot at correction. Magic did not take the AIDS test. He would have been too busy, too macho and maybe too scared. Magic had to take the insurance exam to play basketball. In taking that exam, they detected HIV.

The bad news for him was that he was humiliated, embarrassed and had to stop playing basketball. The good news was early detection meant he could start getting treatment and he could use his persona as a source of education. He really turned a deadly minus into a plus. He's alive because of one thing . . . early detection.

That's why for me the most important achievement of Indiana Black Expo is not the sellout audiences enjoying the fall classic football game and battle of the bands. It's not the 95,000 drawn to the Music Heritage Festival during the summer celebration. It's not the hundreds of thousands of people filing through the turnstiles to patronize the rows and rows of vendors and exhibitors each year. The Health Fair is the most important Expo function.

A part of me always realized the truth even though I never acted like it when it came to my own life. Nonetheless it remains true. Nothing is more important than health. None of the many offerings we have at our disposal from day to day can be enjoyed without being physically capable of accessing them. The health fair is the most important Expo function. I've always known it and I've always felt it. Now, for me, it has new meaning and offers new hope.

It offers hope that maybe someone without a family doctor, without life insurance, without any information on the risk of prostate cancer—or any of the other life-threatening diseases for which testing is offered at the Summer Celebration health fair—

will make his or her way into the event this year or next and take the tests.

It offers hope that if a person's examination results are positive that person will get early treatment. Maybe, as a result, that person will get a second chance at a longer, better quality of life.

What IBE activity could possibly provide more gratification?

Chapter Three

PLAYING DOCTOR

IGNORING THE EARLY WARNING SIGNS OF A POTENTIAL KILLER

The last thing any man should do is play doctor with his health.

Just because you feel a twinge in your chest doesn't mean you're having a heart attack. If you're a person who rarely gets sick, then you probably don't take mild symptoms too seriously.

I wasn't any different. I knew very little about prostate cancer. I was unaware that it is the most common form of cancer among American men and that most cases occur among men over fifty (I was fifty-four when first diagnosed). It never occurred to me that I was only one of almost 180,000 new cases in 2002. Sadly, over 32,000 men died from the disease that same year.

The American Cancer Society cites two particular facts that should be a wake-up call for every black man in America.

- First, African American males who are diagnosed with prostate cancer are more likely to be in the advanced stages of the disease. (In my case, the statistic was true.

My diagnosis revealed that my cancer was in the most advanced stage.)
- Second, for reasons yet unknown to medical experts, the mortality rate for African American men with prostate cancer is more than twice that of white men.

Knowledge of my family health history had never been a priority for me. It should have been. Genetics play an important role in establishing the probability of getting prostate cancer. Scientists think that the disease may cluster in some families. They think that men with a family history of prostate cancer have an increased risk for developing prostate cancer themselves. The risk spirals upward as the total number of affected family members increases.

Cancer runs in my family. My grandmother died of skin cancer. Both my mother and sister are breast cancer survivors. When I thought about it, I mistakenly concluded that these relatives were all women and their illnesses had nothing to do with me. My father had heart problems that resulted in bypass surgery. He also has high blood pressure. But he didn't have cancer so I didn't think it was a threat.

All of this was the product of foolish thinking and ignorance. Somehow I never knew, or conveniently forgot, that my mother's two brothers—Jimmy and Harry—both had prostate cancer.

No one should go through life worrying about dying. There are no percentages in becoming preoccupied with the prospect of getting sick while you're feeling well. Fear can be as crippling as an actual affliction. But in retrospect, I should have been more wary of the possibilities; more alert to my body.

Somewhere along the line, an alarm should have sounded in my head to signal the need for caution. It never happened. I was too busy with a daily schedule that started before dawn and stretched into the night. It's hard to pause long enough to deal with personal health issues when you're always on the go.

Many men today use the same twisted logic. We are too busy to give needed attention to health care because we feel great and look to be in relatively good shape. Warning: If we don't change our priorities—the consequences may be deadly.

Suddenly, the health concern that ranked lowest on my "to do" list before my diagnosis is just about the only thing I have time for any more; my number one priority, the ominous presence of every waking hour. The same issue of personal health that seemed so negligible for so long has become my consuming, relentless preoccupation.

Other things that once meant so much have become trivial. It's hard to adjust to being sick when you've managed to live a relatively healthy life. Of course, there were a few colds in winter and a bout with bronchitis once but that was it for me for a long time. It was so easy to be lulled into thinking that cancer would never happen to me. Like most men, I went about my business, never admitting I might be vulnerable.

Even when your body gives you a hint that something is awry, it's easier to play doctor and rule out the chances of those symptoms signaling anything serious. That's the advantage of being your own doctor, your bedside manner is impeccable and the diagnosis is always favorable. The mind can easily dupe a person into a feeling of invincibility.

The truth is, most of us don't want to know that we have a problem—as if ignorance will make it go away. Fear of the unknown can be debilitating. Fear can make the best thinkers use the worst judgment. It can make men who generously offer a spiritual harbor to others in distress drift aimlessly in their own ocean of denial, apprehension and rationalization.

As your own doctor, you consult with close friends or relatives about the aches and pains that you believe to be of minimal consequence. I was close enough to individuals in the medical community to get telephone consultation even without the benefit of an exam.

Tell doctors only what you want them to know and it's more likely that they will tell you just what you want to hear. I was able to get my physician friends to give me prescriptions for the nagging symptoms I was experiencing without them ever dealing with the actual illness. At other times, I settled for homespun remedies or over-the-counter drugs that folks outside of the medical profession insisted would make the pain go away.

I did whatever was possible to avoid facing reality. The delay was costly.

My earliest sign of trouble came in 1999, when it became increasingly difficult for me to achieve and maintain an erection. The thought of a urinary or prostate infection crossed my mind. But in my mode of self-diagnosis, I attributed my lack of sexual performance to aging and too much alcohol. If I cut back on drinking, I thought, my virility would return to form.

Only after allowing the problems to get worse for a year did I finally consult my primary care physician. After a routine physical, he told me that I was suffering from a prostate infection, which was common for men my age. No prostate-specific antigen (PSA) blood test, or digital rectal exam (DRE) was administered.

My problems worsened. There was no relief. Yet, I continued to ignore the need for a second opinion throughout the following year. Only after my symptoms: pain, fatigue, and just not feeling well, reached a point at which I could take it no longer did I consent to an office visit with a new doctor. He checked my PSA. The normal range for the test is 0 to 4. My PSA was an astronomical 172.3! The doctor ordered me to see a urologist immediately.

Instead, I delayed again, and further delayed the inevitable. Why did I delay? I can't explain it easily. Maybe it was fear. Sometimes otherwise intelligent men just do the wrong thing even though they know better.

I continued to experience the severe symptoms of prostate cancer.

Every man should know how to identify some of these early warning signs. They include

- Frequent urination
- Inability to urinate
- Trouble starting or holding back the flow, weak or interrupted flow
- Painful or burning during urination, blood in the urine or semen
- Impotence
- Painful ejaculation
- Frequent pain or stiffness in the lower back, pelvic, hips or upper thighs

Men need not always fear the worst if they have any of these symptoms. While they can be symptoms of cancer, medical experts say they are more often symptoms of non-cancerous enlargement of the prostate. The way it works is this: As men get older, their prostate may grow larger and block the flow of urine or interfere with sexual function. This common condition is called benign prostatic hyperplasia (BPH). It is not cancer, but can cause many of the same symptoms of prostate cancer. Although BPH may not be life threatening, it may require treatment with medicine or surgery to relieve symptoms.

Sometimes a man can get lost in the possibilities. Sometimes the worst fears are unfounded—no matter how many signs may point in a single direction. And sometimes our hopes are dashed when it is revealed that our worst fears are coming true.

The bottom line is truth is your only weapon.

Those who insist that they never play doctor, who immediately seek medical attention whenever something goes wrong or doesn't feel right,—should not develop a false sense of security. Prostate cancer can occur and advance in men with no symptoms at all. There's just no way of determining the truth until you step up and take the tests.

Even with PSA results off the charts, for reasons I can't explain, I still refused to accept the gravity of the situation. It would be another five months before I took the next step.

During that waiting period—on a chilly night in March at home—I remember awakening in the dark with severe pains in my hips and ribs. At first I tried, but was unable, to get out of bed. I finally rolled out of bed in tears and practically had to crawl to the bathroom. I didn't want to disturb my son who was sleeping.

A trip to the emergency room would have been the most logical course to take but instead I chose to go through an agonizing night, tossing restlessly in bed throughout the ordeal. Small consolation came the next day as the pain subsided to a level at which I was able to function. Again, the morbid dread of the unknown forced me into downplaying this excruciating experience as just another single incident.

I guess I thought that ignoring or minimizing the problem might make it go away. So whenever there was a slight discomfort, I chose to clench my jaws and bear the pain. Whenever there was a grinding pressure or intense pain, it was dismissed as a passing feeling . . . no cause for alarm.

My ill-conceived strategy seemed to work most of the time until May, 2002—five months after the astounding PSA level was detected. In that usually bright month, I was referred to a sports medicine doctor. I complained that the pain in my right hip was unlike anything I had ever felt. Ever the "play doctor," I suggested arthritis. Unaware of my PSA, the sports medicine doctor took X-rays and diagnosed bursitis. He prescribed anti-inflammatory medication.

I knew better. It was just another subliminal delaying tactic. The longer you avoid the whole truth, the longer it takes medical people to accurately pinpoint the problem. I should have mentioned the PSA results, and all my other symptoms.

It was a chess game with my life at stake. The message to all of my caretakers was "help me if you can." I wasn't willing to make any contribution to the effort. I may even have felt a bizarre sense of accomplishment that I could throw off the doctors' diagnosis of my problem. But in the game of denial and deception, the winner is the loser.

I knew that the sports medicine doctor's prescription of anti-inflammatory drugs and physical therapy was a waste of time.

After all, he was working without all of the facts. But it bought me a little more time to try and outrun my fate, refusing to accept the fact that there was no escape.

The chess game lasted only two weeks. After the visit to the sports medicine doctor, the pain increased. When I couldn't take it any longer I returned to my general practitioner on May 27, 2002, with an intolerable throbbing in my hip, lower back and pelvis. By then the intense discomfort in my stomach and ribs folded me into a fetal position on the examination table. The next day, a CAT scan and other laboratory tests were administered at St. Vincent Hospital in Indianapolis. The results came two days later. I had cancer. I was referred to Dr. Andrew Moore, a leading urologist in the Indianapolis area. He scheduled a biopsy and, afterwards, a consultation.

My mother, sister, significant other and executive assistant—the people I cherished most in life—were with me when the doctor told me I was suffering from prostatic carcinoma with metastatic disease in the ribs and the lymph nodes. Put simply, I had prostate cancer in its most advanced stage; it had already begun to spread throughout my body. After those startling results.

The severity of prostate cancer, like many other cancers, is specified by the stage it is in when diagnosed. Prostate cancer is specified in four stages, from most treatable to least treatable. The stages are:

- Stage 1 and 2. Early prostate cancer is localized to the prostate gland and is highly treatable.
- Stage 3. The cancer is advanced outside the prostate, but localized in nearby tissues.

- Stage 4. The prostate cancer has spread to other organs or tissue.

I had Stage 4 prostatic carcinoma with metastatic disease. Hormone therapy and estrogen were prescribed. My biggest frustration is knowing that if I had done the right thing earlier, my chances of recovery would be much greater.

As we sat in the doctor's office, my mind wandered as I thought about my condition even as the doctor fielded a flurry of questions from Kathy and Valerie. The doctor sought the right words to explain the critical diagnosis and possibilities to my family members and friends.

He told them that my cancer couldn't be cured, that the most we could hope for would be to contain it and that there was no way of knowing how much time I had left to live. Naturally, it made me cry.

Yet, through the tears, gloom and anxiety of that session, my state of mind was reduced to one concern—the inability to have sex.

Not being able to achieve or maintain an erection can disturb a man, married or single. The possibility of sacrificing sexual prowess for the rest of my life seemed unimaginable.

The reality of impotency in many sufferers of prostate cancer is probably one of the primary obstacles in the campaign to persuade more African American men to confess their symptoms, get tested and seek timely treatment. The self-imposed silence that results from the sense of "shame" and "weakness" men feel also denies them the ability to network with others in the same situation.

The silence, unfortunately, is a man thing.

My treatment started immediately. The first phases of the treatment included hormone therapy, with two drugs called Casodex® and Lupron-Depot®. These drugs were prescribed to lower the level of testosterone that feeds the cancer cells. From my standpoint, their impact was about the same as castration, only by chemical means. Without adequate testosterone, there would be virtually no chance for me to have an erection.

Strangely, not even the threat of death chilled me to the bone as much as the prospect of never being able to make love again. That was my first and most demoralizing reaction—the tremendous sense of loss and inadequacy in contemplating never having sex again. Let's face it, sex is pivotal in much of our society and commands a disproportionate amount of the attention of men of all races. It's everywhere in the media and often in our minds.

Right or wrong, the ability to perform sexually has traditionally been equated with manhood in the thoughts, if not the words, of many Americans. Without the ability to make love, I was essentially facing the prospect—at least from my distorted perspective at the time—of being reduced to less than a man.

It was a month or more before I summoned the courage to look at my position truthfully. My perspective broadened as I reflected on where I had come from, the place in which I found myself, and where I might be heading. Thinking it all through, it dawned on me that my attitude about sex was not only shallow, but selfish.

In rethinking my plight, I began to realize that in dealing with prostate cancer I was confronting life or death, living or dying. A question came to me as I thought about my beautiful children, caring family, and compassionate lady. It was a simple question, yet startling in its clarity: What price, I asked myself, is too high to pay for the blessing of another God-given day?

It dawned on me then that sex is just a part of life—not the essence of life. Sex is only one form of intimacy. Those who have to do without it need only to explore other forms.

The thought of how blessed I am struck me. The realization of the number of people I have helped and have yet to help came to mind. Then it was all clear. So much good could come out of my unfortunate reality if I regained my focus and offered whatever influence I might have to benefit people who may be touched, enlightened, encouraged or enriched through sharing my experience.

There would be many mountains to climb. Laboratory tests on July 25, 2002 confirmed that the cancer had spread to my bones.

Coping with the immediate side effects of the initial cancer-fighting treatment and medication is a constant challenge. Some of the side-effects of my treatment were:

- Impotence
- Hot- flashes
- Breast enlargement
- Weight gain
- Depression

The symptoms made it kind of touchy for me when encountering people in public who couldn't detect any outward changes in me. Months after treatment began, people would come up to me, surprised that I still looked the picture of health. What they really meant was that I hadn't lost weight like other cancer victims they've known. These people were just unaware that with prostate cancer men may lose weight or gain weight. The side effects of the treatment I was receiving over a two-month period during the fall of 2002 actually caused me to gain sixteen pounds. So the words that people meant as a compliment were of no comfort. I just learned to accept the spirit of their concern.

Every day I fought that melancholy temperament that made me a stranger to myself. I've always been an emotional person, but never depressed. Personal or professional setbacks were only challenges for me to find new ways to reach my goals.

Whenever I asked someone for anything and they said "no," I just concluded that either they didn't understand the question or it should have been stated differently. I am that irrepressible spirit, eternal optimist, dreamer. My enthusiasm has always been buoyed by my faith in God and reaffirmed by the long list of successful ventures I have been blessed to work on.

Yet in the wake of my prostate cancer treatment, I had an unrelenting sense of emptiness.

I frequently found myself in crowds of friends and well-wishing strangers—and coped by putting on the best possible face, the most upbeat front that could be mustered. My response was always the lie that I was doing fine.

The truth is that some days are more manageable than others. Most days you just pray for deliverance, for the strength to endure. There were times when I was overcome with the feeling that I would rather be dead than bear such pain. Moments of weakness are unavoidable when you are faced with indescribable pain. But the despair doesn't linger.

Aside from the pain, there were side effects of the treatment that were less hurtful but equally agitating. The advent of hot flashes, for example, is something that a man really can't prepare for before it happens. Just imagine your body overheating uncontrollably five or six times a day. It gives you a greater appreciation of what women go through on a regular basis.

Women suffer the joy and pain of childbirth along with myriad health challenges. Measuring the pain tolerance of men to that of women is comparing the pop of a firecracker with the deafening blast of a sonic boom. "Menopause" is just another word in the dictionary for most men. While some make a token effort to research and empathize with their mates, in most cases, men feel that it's enough for them to show tolerance as women 'go through the change.' It's difficult for men to relate. Few even try.

Sometimes nature has a way of putting the proverbial shoe on the other foot. I've learned the hard way. Even in the biting cold of winter, I find myself having to sleep with both a ceiling fan and a floor fan on trying to cool the hot flashes that I experience throughout the night.

At one point, I continued going to my office at Expo. It was embarrassing whenever I'd break out into a sweat—right in the middle of a business meeting—from the implosion of my body heat.

All of my life it has been important for me to respect women. If men developed a greater capacity to appreciate the magnificent natural strength women possess, the spiritual foundation they lay for our society and the source of sustenance they provide when our own manhood is under-nourished, we would rise for spontaneous ovations at the very thought of womanhood.

Ultimately, men with prostate cancer will know they are blessed if they have any semblance of the kind of mother, sister and soul mate that I have had to help me through my crisis.

My mother's and sister's journeys on a path similar to mine provides a key aid in my struggle to cope. Little did I know, as I prayed at their bedsides and nursed them, that the roles would soon be reversed.

Solemn but subdued is the manner in which I accept my fate regarding impotence. The depression that was at one point so consuming was thankfully short-lived. Even the effects of the hormone treatment have diminished in my mind to necessary evils.

Scripture affirms that God puts no more on us than he knows we can bear. Even when we doubt ourselves, He knows. Even when others become skeptical, He knows. So though the burden may not feel lighter, knowledge of the power of the Word makes it easier to bear.

The most difficult aspect I had to reconcile was the nagging question of 'what might have been.'

Think about it. Through early and regular examination, there can only be two consequences. Either you confirm your worst fears but improve the chances for effective treatment, or you have your fears dispelled by professional, medical affirmation that you don't have prostate cancer. It's a win-win situation. The only losing proposition is to continue functioning in the dark—choosing not to take care of business—running the risk of making the situation worse by doing nothing about it.

Because my faith is unflappable, I pray the Lord will forgive my unwillingness to take His precious gift of life more seriously and will use me as an example—to shine a light for others. African American men must be reminded that the Almighty works through the hands and minds of His creations—the surgeons, general practitioners, urologists, oncologists, and radiologists He blessed with expertise and talent.

It is up to each of us to access all that is available to reap those blessings.

It would be foolhardy to weave a speeding car recklessly through traffic on a busy interstate while praying that we be protected from getting struck by another vehicle. Prayer requires responsibility. Faith requires works. If a man is aware of his need to get professional attention, to address a potentially serious health concern, but still refuses to take the necessary steps, it reflects disobedience, for which consequences may be grave.

Much is left to chance—even under the best conditions, when a man is diagnosed with prostate cancer. The process doesn't need to be further complicated by the temptation for us to play doctor.

CHAPTER FOUR

A WOMAN'S TOUCH

THE POWER OF WIVES, LOVERS, MOTHERS, DAUGHTERS AND FRIENDS

Cancer spreads beyond the body of the patient. People who care about the victims suffer too. I was overcome with that compelling sense of empathy when my sister, Kathy, was diagnosed with breast cancer. An eerie sense of déjà vu occurred when my mother became afflicted with the same disease.

Both of them fought and survived their physical challenges. Though there is precious little anyone can actually do to affect the outcome, the spiritual and moral imperative is to always be there for the people in your life. It warms my heart during the darkest hours to know that my mother and sister are companions through my ordeal.

A popular country and western song belts out the lyric title, "Stand by Your Man." There may be no more important time for a woman to do just that than when he is stricken. Impotence is the one obvious concern men have when they suffer prostate cancer. But it goes so much deeper than that. Some people begin to question their sense of worth, and lose their resolve to fight. A woman's touch can bring a man's dying spirit back to life. When things look bleak and the body gets weak, the most potent antidote is for that special someone to speak.

Valerie Parker is the mother of my eight-year-old daughter, Shakara. She is also an articulate, intelligent, compassionate, accomplished career woman in Indianapolis. She is the woman in my life. Before my diagnosis, we decided to get married. When prostate cancer was discovered in its most advanced stages, I backed off, though she was still willing. While I was gratified by the sacrifice she was willing to make, it's impossible for me to ignore or downplay the point that I may be incapable of fulfilling her sexual desires.

It's important to me to share some of the thoughts of the women close to me, the ones most deeply affected by my condition. If you are a man who doesn't have prostate cancer, the thoughts of these wonderful women may help you see how you risk hurting others by not being examined regularly. If you already have prostate cancer, the revealing expressions of these women will be helpful and even heartening.

If you happen to be a female reader, these comments are offered in the hope that they will reinforce how important it is for you to urge the men that you care about to stop making excuses and put their health first.

Here are Valerie's own words:

When Charles first shared his symptoms with me in September of 1999, he was concerned that all was not well. However, Charles decided that he didn't want to rush to conclusions, so he put off going to a doctor, figuring that he could sort of wait it out. He continued with his hectic work schedule. That included honoring speaking engagements, attending his daughter and son's extra-curricular events, and being there whenever someone called—as he had always been.

It's upsetting, to say the least, watching your man deal with burning urination, anxiety, irregular heartbeats, light-headedness, fluid retention, the inability to achieve or maintain an erection and a relentless overall funk.

Charles was conscious of what his body was saying but conveniently attributed symptoms to all the wrong things. He refused to give in to the possibility that a doctor's visit was in order. So unchecked, conditions worsened. When Charles finally gave in and went for a physical in December, 1999, his blood pressure was life-threateningly high. He was immediately hospitalized. For the first time in his life, Charles was diagnosed with high blood pressure. After days of hospitalization and a battery of tests, he was released with a new prescription to keep the blood pressure under control. Within a week after his release, the symptoms of what had earlier been diagnosed as prostate infection returned and intensified. He also began to feel severe pelvic pain. But rather than digging deeper for the causes, Charles spent all of the year 2000 taking medication to alleviate the misery. I never stopped pleading for him to get more tests.

Charles's thoughts were calmed by his physician's diagnosis. Though an examination revealed that Charles's prostate was enlarged, his doctor said that such ailments were common and highly treatable among men over fifty. That doctor had done a digital rectal exam but had never given Charles a PSA test. Throughout the rest of that year, Charles refused to seek a second opinion.

There was a sense of renewed hope in 2001 when Charles started out the year seeming to feel a lot better. His blood pressure had sta-

bilized and he had resumed his regular workout schedule. Though symptoms continued in some measure, they seemed to be manageable with regular dosages of Levaquin. The optimism was short-lived. By May of 2001, Charles began to feel poorly again.

While having no idea that his condition might be terminal, Charles appeared willing to accept that his poor health was chronic and he would have to face it from now on. It tore me apart to watch the vicious attacks and see that he wasn't getting any better.

By the end of 2001, the only comfortable sleeping position for Charles was sitting up. I remember watching him try to doze in an upright position on Christmas Eve. I told myself that something was seriously wrong and that it was time to begin urging him to go to the doctor again.

Often men of power, who are accustomed to calling the shots, are their own worst enemies. I believe there are a number of reasons Charles refused to seek answers for so long. For a majority of men, going to the doctor is simply not on the priority list. When he first experienced symptoms, he had no immediate concern because he felt that he could self-diagnose the problem away.

Taking time from a full schedule to get a check-up threatened to deprive him of at least one of the activities he enjoyed so much more. First, there was his beloved IBE, then the unending devotion to being active in the education and activities of his two youngest children. Then he was busy going to Pacer and Colts games, teeing it up on the golf course, making personal appearances and playing trivia games with a group of teachers who met regularly at a restaurant a few blocks from his home.

Charles was also devout about his physical conditioning regimen. It began when he lost more than a hundred pounds by changing his eating habits and faithfully sticking to a strict workout schedule.

With the help of a trainer, Charles developed an athletic chest and a 'six pack' abdomen. He was proud of the results. His conditioning plan made no provision for catastrophic illness. Looking back, it seems ironic that the same emphasis placed on the outside of the body wasn't focused within.

But the pain Charles was going through simply would not ebb. Anticipating resistance to my unending "encouragement" for my stubborn soul mate to get a second opinion, I was willing, and ready, to endure his anger. I had reached the conclusion that he was worth the fight.

Soon after the holidays, I approached him when he was clearly not at his best and gently said that something was seriously wrong, something beyond what his doctors told him. I said that we needed to know the whole truth. Charles spoke quietly, without looking up, saying only, 'Make the appointment.' I did and we went to a different doctor in January, 2002.

For the first time, Charles took the PSA test. Given his astronomically high PSA level of 172.3, it was clear that this was not the result of an enlarged prostate. The diagnosis of cancer was imminent and it was mortifying. Incredibly, in the wake of his PSA, it took five months for Charles to get to the urologist!

On May 27, 2002, in the wake of intense pain, Charles made a trip to Dr. Thomas Petrin's office. Dr. Petrin ordered a CAT scan in addition to another PSA test. Two days later, the results were in. There was cancer in the lymph nodes and the PSA had risen a few points. It was now 175. Dr. Petrin suspected that the area of the body where the cancer originally started was the prostate. Charles was immediately referred to his urologist, Dr. Andrew Moore, for further examination.

A biopsy of the prostate was scheduled and performed June 10,

2002. The results were absolutely devastating. I was truly sick about it. All I could think about was that I loved this man. It wasn't fair to him, to me, to his children or family. The diagnosis was prostatic carcinoma with metastatic disease involving the ribs and lymph nodes. Charles was told that his cancer was diagnosed at the most advanced stage and it was suspected that it had also spread. A bone scan along with additional tests would be scheduled.

I watched him. I held his hand. And as I sat there and listened to Dr. Moore, I began to pray silently because I knew God would see us through even this.

I was extremely concerned not only about Charles's physical outlook but his emotional outlook as well. Here is a man who has always been in charge. In the past, he would push himself to the limit and always land on his feet. He is strong, and independent. He's also a man who makes things happen. He relished the role of leadership, of taking risks, of making decisions. It worried me to think how he might cope with the prospect of severe physical limitations beyond his control.

There was a part of me that wanted to fix it. But I began to accept what I already had known in my heart—that Charles was really sick and I couldn't make it go away. It filled me with sadness and anger. I was sad realizing that home remedies and prescription drugs were unable to control the disease.

I was angry that Charles had not gone in for treatment earlier; angry because he refused to get a second opinion, and angry that through all of his suffering, he didn't seem serious enough about getting to the root of his problem. I was angry that the first physician didn't give him a more thorough examination, and that he didn't demand more tests after Charles didn't improve from the medication he prescribed.

There were times when I was afraid that whatever Charles was experiencing physically was getting the best of him. I recognized that the way he was feeling was not always something he wanted to talk about.

So I was careful not to react but to respond, not to pry but to listen, not to press for decisions but simply to share what I thought were viable options. I was careful to approach him only when the time was right, when he seemed open, when he seemed in search of answers. Charles continued trying to function normally in an effort to focus on anything but the physical challenge he was facing.

In the beginning, the realization of our fears was difficult to handle. I felt Charles was riveted with an overwhelming desire for answers to his questions. And for the first time, I felt very strongly his fear and shared that same fear. We were both careful not to speak fear into existence. We both chose to just deal with the experience very quietly as we continued the search for answers.

In the end, the one thing that concerned me most was his reaction to the sexual aspect of prostate cancer. It was important to me that he not let impotence tear him apart. I wanted to show him that there were so many ways to display love and intimacy other than making love.

It seemed that with every episode of symptoms, Charles's desire for intimacy decreased. Like many women, my first thought was that his lack of attention was the result of a loss of interest in me. Even though he constantly reassured me that I wasn't the problem, there were times when the words spoken were difficult to believe.

The awkwardness wasn't all about me. I saw how agonizing it was for Charles not to be able to function as he always had in the past. Like too many men, he equated sex with manhood. In an effort to deny the seriousness of his dysfunction, he minimized the problem, blaming it on drinking. Trying to avoid reality, he turned to Viagra.

The drug delivered as advertised. But it was nothing more than a short-term fix, a temporary alternative, not a lasting solution. The medicaton wasn't designed to cure cancer.

Eventually, the limitations of Charles's health became very real to him. Rather than face the consequences of his changing body, he decided not to talk about it. He denied the problem and ignored the situation. Trying to be supportive, I wasn't sure if I should bring it up or not.

For a while, we kept silent on the subject, hoping in our minds that we would eventually get past it. After several months of inaction—and no conversation about our love life—we decided to express to each other how we felt. Our quiet, soulful discussions were as passionate as any sexual encounter imaginable. We learned the pleasures of being inside of each other's thoughts—not just our bodies.

What he revealed taught me that sexual dysfunction has to be one of the most difficult problems for any man to confront. I don't think that Charles felt as deficient as much as he felt defective. There were times when I didn't know the right words to say. I had to learn to accept that sometimes nothing that I could say was enough. And yet men need our words of comfort, reassurance and validation.

In our most revealing 'quiet moments,' Charles told me that the hardest part about being unable to perform sexual intercourse was that physical intimacy was the only way he knew to express intimacy. I told him that the simple honesty of sharing our deepest thoughts was romantic and that there could be nothing more erotic than sharing each other's joy and pain.

Sometimes I worried that my best efforts at comforting conversation wouldn't last when we weren't in each other's company—that for the first time, I couldn't just kiss the pain away. But in time

Charles grew more self-assured and comfortable with his situation. He'd realized how much more there is to life and love. When I saw that, I knew that he had reached a new level of understanding.

For the first time, not only did he accept his challenge but he didn't care if the world knew about it. He wanted to let the community know what he was going through as a warning for other men to get checked out.

When Charles first approached me about his decision to make his health public, I had mixed emotions. Everything seemed to be happening so fast. I had my doubts about his strategy. Then, in the quiet of one night, as I sat alone with my thoughts and my God, I prayed for understanding, strength, grace and mercy. I fought my feelings that centered on the possible negative impact such publicity might have on his children and me. I wondered why he was so driven to sacrifice so much.

Time passed without word on the proposal to go public. I thought he had dropped the notion and I sure wasn't planning on mentioning the idea again. A short while later, he called me one Saturday morning and told me to go on the Internet and look up the Indianapolis Star. *I did. Not only was there a large news article about Charles battling prostate cancer but it was right across the top of the front page.*

To say I was shocked would be an understatement. But the article was tasteful and well written. The reporters had interviewed him and included general facts and statistics on prostate cancer—particularly relating to African American men. I didn't telephone Charles right away. I needed time to sort out my true feelings.

I really needed to assess my emotions as well as my thoughts before talking to Charles about his decision to go public. On the one hand, I recognized that more people knowing about his illness would mean more people praying for his recovery. It also seemed logical that revealing the facts would discourage vicious rumors and unkind, uninformed rumors about Charles's health issues.

Eventually, it came to me that it wasn't really about the children or me. It was about Charles's healing. In his estimation, going forward openly and truthfully was the first major step toward his victory. It became clear that he was not only committed to recovery, but to educating and informing others about prostate cancer. His actions affirmed that he had accepted the illness, acknowledged the journey ahead, and was prepared to meet the challenge.

After those thoughts came to me, I found a peace about the entire ordeal. When Charles and I talked, I assured him that he had my unwavering support. What he has decided to do serves as advocacy for the health of black men across this country. In the final analysis, if you know Charles, you know he really had no choice. It is testament to his uncompromising devotion to helping others at any personal sacrifice. I should've known all along that he had no choice.

Through the peaks and valleys of my tribulations, there is nothing that Valerie hasn't done to make my burden lighter. I don't even want to imagine what going through this would be like without her. To have someone who can light up my life like Valerie is a magnificent blessing.

Everyone has a personal life and a business side. While Valerie sustains the former, Lynna Townsend sustains the latter. She is a pure gem.

Lynna is more than just my secretary and personal assistant. She is one of my closest friends and has been for years. I can tell her everything. In my absence, I trust her to be my voice. Since cancer has limited my ability to get into the office, a computer

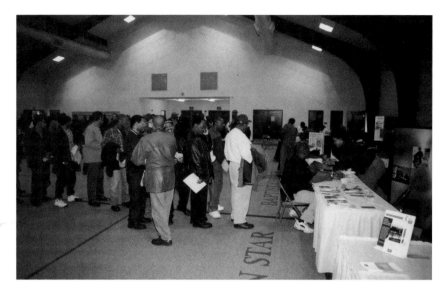

Eastern Star Church, 2003 Men's Health Fair

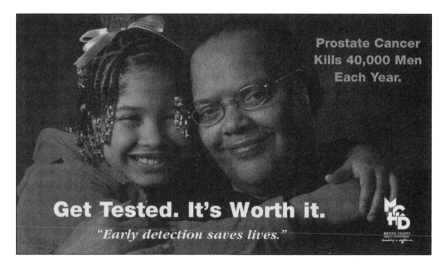

Rev. Williams and his daughter Shakara promoting prostate
awareness and screening.

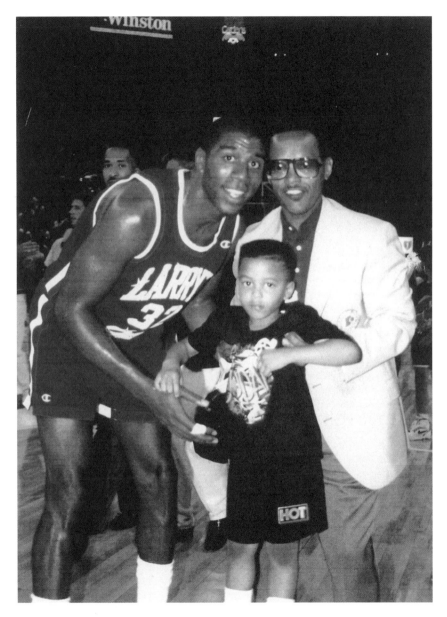

"Magic" Johnson, Charles Williams, Jr. and Rev. Charles Williams.

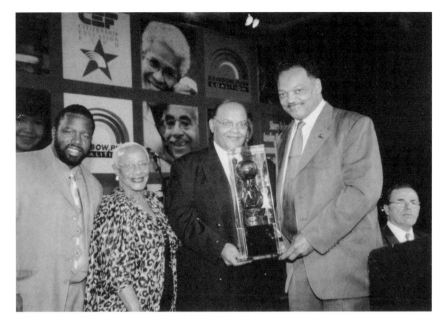

Rev. Jesse Jackson presenting an award from Operation PUSH to Rev. Williams. Also pictured are Rev. James Meeks (left) and Rev. Willie Barrow (right)

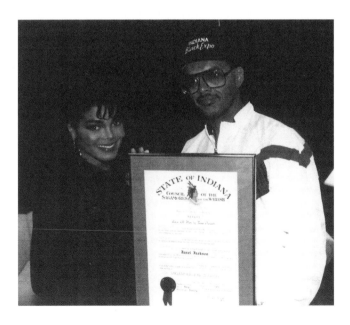

Rev. Williams with Janet Jackson

(photo by Beverly Swanagan © 2002)

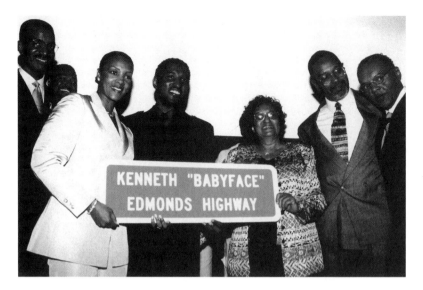

Moses Brewer, Vivica Fox, Kenneth "Babyface" Edmonds, Barbara Edmonds, Addison T. Simpson, and Rev. Charles Williams at the "renaming" of the Kenneth "Babyface" Edmonds Highway

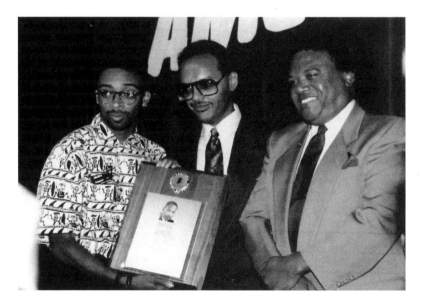

Spike Lee, Rev. Williams, and State Representative William Crawford

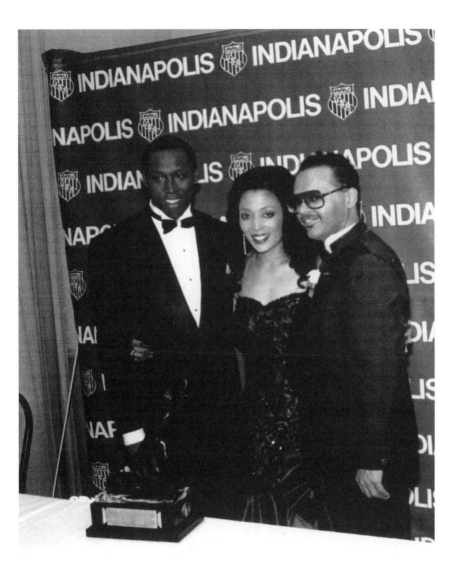

Al Joyner, Florence Griffith Joyner, and Rev. Williams

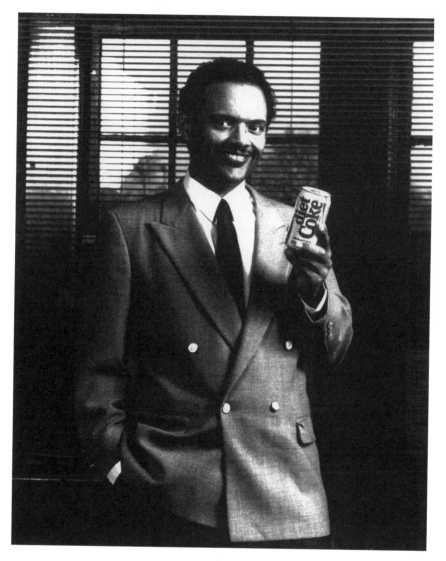

Reverend Charles Williams

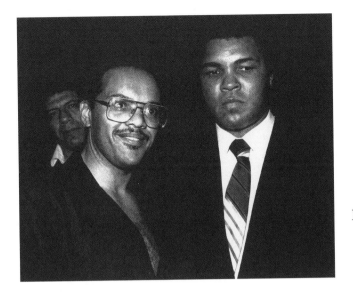

Rev. Williams
and
Muhammad
Ali

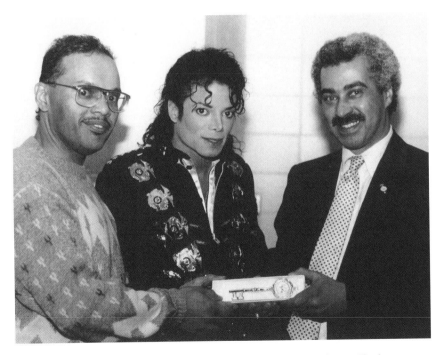

Rev. Charles Williams, Michael Jackson, and Joe Slash

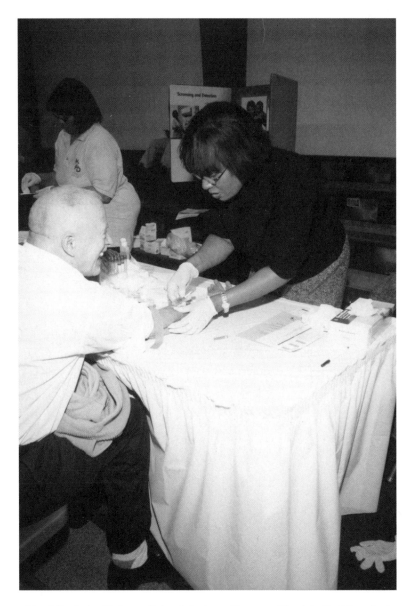

Dr. Virginia Caine of the Marion County Health & Hospital Corporation doing a PSA screening.

has been set up for me at home so I can continue working even though I can't get into my office every day. The technology creates a solution. Lynna makes it happen.

To give you an idea of how important Lynna is in my life, when my mother, sister and Valerie joined me at Dr. Andrew Moore's office to hear my diagnosis, Lynna was also there. She is another one of the very special women in my life who brings a unique perspective to my health concerns. Some of Lynna's thoughts help shed light on this disease.

Reverend Charles Williams is my lil' boss and I love him. These past few years have been difficult for me because we are so close. I have known about his illness since 2000. There were so many different health problems that kept cropping up and he would always attribute them to something minor. In the back of my mind I always knew that things just weren't adding up.

Charles would be sick and call some of his doctor friends to get a self-diagnosed prescription. Either someone on the staff or I would pick it up from the pharmacy. Not once did Charles have a complete check up. He was always too busy.

Being on the board of Winona Memorial Hospital, any time Charles wasn't feeling well, he could go to the Fast Care service there and they would take him right in. For two years, my lil' boss was dealing with some personal issues and a lot of craziness on the job. All of it left him in a somber mood.

Looking back, I'm convinced that the stress of being the Reverend Charles Williams was definitely a factor. He wasn't himself most of the time. I can't pinpoint the time at which Charles got cancer. But I know from the progression of symptoms, it didn't just happen overnight.

My most vivid recollection of the appointment with Dr. Andrew Moore was how prepared Val and Kathy were. They had done their homework on prostate cancer and were firing questions at the doctor. All I could think to ask was whether Charles would be in too much pain to drive.

Charles didn't like the question and told me to 'shut up.' I remember thinking, he must feel better because that was more like his old self. It was only wishful thinking. Charles was ill. And he wasn't the only one angry during the meeting with the doctor. The rest of us were incensed that Charles' friends in the medical profession pacified him all of those years instead of forcing him to get examined.

Charles always dreaded the prostate exam because others told him how uncomfortable they were when the doctor stuck a finger up the rectum. I guess it's a man thing. One of the happiest and saddest days of my life was when my lil' boss was finally talked into going to the doctor. Time lost was costly.

But Charles has determination like few people you will ever meet. He's been at this place in his life many times before—when people told him what couldn't be done. With the help of God, he always managed to overcome adversity. Why should this fight be any different? I am taking his illness one day at a time. My most important duty is to make sure that he keeps his medical appointments. Other than that, I just want to be there for my lil' boss."

The love of the women in my life is like a breath of fresh air. Armed with their affirmations, prayers and the word of God, my fight is one I will win.

Every woman has a relationship with at least one man. It may be a father, son, brother, cousin, uncle, nephew, neighbor, colleague, husband, lover or friend. Whatever the association, it is important for women to encourage their men to undergo prostate testing early and regularly, each year. That message can't be repeated enough, especially among African Americans.

Prostate cancer isn't a "for men only" crisis. It can only be conquered if women play a role. Every man needs a woman's touch. Even if the man is stubborn, don't give up. Be relentless. It's worth the trouble.

CHAPTER FIVE

BLIZZARD IN SUMMER

FACING THE REALITY OF
THE "C" WORD

In the early stages of my battle with prostate cancer, I was caught up in my own emotions and self-pity. It's so easy to feel sorry for yourself when you are the victim of a terminal illness. I had to remind myself that there are hundreds of thousands of men just like me.

Men with prostate cancer eventually have to face the reality of the "C" word and rise above it. We have to know what God wants us to do and then follow His command.

In doing our part, we must recognize that faith without works is meaningless. We can't just sit back and wait on the Lord to do all of the work. In that spirit, I had to learn how not to sigh and moan about what a terrible thing this is to have happened to me. Instead, I had to become active in the fight for my life. The first step was to begin exploring all the different courses of treatment and to get as much information about the disease as possible.

Kathy and Valerie understood this need from the beginning. They amassed a huge amount of information on prostate cancer and brought it with them to the doctor's office on the day that my illness was diagnosed. They were so well prepared that they even challenged some of the doctor's initial strategies.

Kathy wanted to know why we couldn't go straight to chemotherapy, skipping treatments in between. She brought with her not only the research documentation, but her own experience with cancer. The doctor insisted on a sequential approach to treatments—with chemotherapy being the last step—and Kathy grudgingly accepted the decision. The important point was that she was able to carry on an intelligent conversation with the physician. That's what all patients should be prepared to do.

On that particular day, I was nowhere near ready to be so pragmatic. The diagnosis had me in a state of shock. I sat silent, numbed by the diagnosis, listening to Kathy, Valerie, and the doctor but not really hearing them. Because the emotion of the moment kept me quiet and distracted, I was glad to have them on my side articulating my case, right from the start. It's a major plus to have supportive and knowledgeable family members with you when you go in to discuss a treatment plan.

Kathy's and Valerie's research provided valuable insights about the different levels of treatment. But there was also a down side. Their research revealed the contradictions within the medical community about the best course of treatment for prostate cancer. Occasionally I thumbed through their material, but I couldn't concentrate on it. Facing the fact that I had cancer was too much of a distraction in itself.

Acknowledging the presence of cancer essentially means facing the possibility of your own death. No matter how "together" you might be in other aspects of your life, this is no easy task. Consider the deep questions surrounding death—questions like:

- What it all means
- What higher purpose can be found in suffering
- How can we overcome the human element of our lives and focus on the spiritual

Obviously, there are no easy answers. In the beginning, I certainly didn't have any. I felt like I was losing my grip and didn't know anything anymore.

Now I'm beyond that period of anxiety, and I've come to terms with my illness. I realize that even as I continue soul-searching for those elusive answers to the big questions, I still have to attend to the immediate need to continue to educate myself about the more tangible problem—my prostate cancer.

Inspired by Kathy and Valerie, I began to do my own research. That is when I began to view myself again as "someone" and not "something." I'm not just another cancer patient. I'm Charles Williams—an individual. Regaining that renewed sense of yourself as an individual allows you to regain and reaffirm your sense of purpose.

A patient will either respond to the "C" word as though he is just waiting to die, or recognize the possibilities and approach the business of treatment and medication with an expectation to live. There's no in between. I choose life. You may never get over the fact that you have prostate cancer. But you have to learn to live with it, and that means understanding it and working in a kind of partnership with your physician.

In medicine, things change every day. I didn't want to just sit back and let the treatment happen to me. I wanted to be involved in, and know about, its risks, its side effects, its potential benefits. But I was able to experience that involvement only when I had reaffirmed a sense of self as an individual and not as a helpless victim.

I found that getting involved requires that the person with prostate cancer:

- become informed enough to ask doctors questions
- collect information from other lay persons familiar with the disease
- wade through the volumes of books and journals available at local medical libraries, and bookstores
- surf the Internet
- dig for any additional resources that will provide the latest possible medical updates

The information's out there. It's accessible, but you have to be diligent in your search. If you have cooperative family members or friends, they will be happy to help you. That way, you won't find the project overwhelming.

After a while, I became absorbed in the research process. I wanted to be prepared and know what to expect—good or bad. I wanted to understand the success rates of the different treatments. In the case of prostate cancer, ignorance is anything but bliss.

Since information fosters understanding, it may also help alleviate fear. Fear isn't good for us. Like stress, it weakens the body. If you are going to fight cancer, you want to be as strong as you can be.

So one of the surprising benefits of my diagnosis was that I learned how to relax for the first time in my life. Strange as it sounds, the concept of relaxation was foreign to me. I was always into something. With Expo, things were constantly at a fever pitch, going straight from one activity to the next. I'd grown accustomed to that pace. If you'd given me the keys to a fabulous condo in Maui, right on the waterfront with no telephones, pagers, cell phones or fax machines, I wouldn't have been able to stand it. Even if surrounded by beautiful palm trees, shimmering white sands, voluptuous island girls, soothing tropical music, delectable entrees, sweet nectar drinks and all the amenities of luxury living, I still would've looked at my watch every few minutes.

Most of my life, I didn't know how to function in such tranquil surroundings. People were always telling me that I needed a vacation, but whenever I went on one it was impossible for me to relax. I couldn't free my mind of business thoughts long enough for my body to feel rejuvenated.

So now, forced by the hands of fate, I've gone from all to nothing; from being a Type "A" overactive individual to being slowed to a crawl by this debilitating illness. Getting involved in research was an important step in making that transition.

As I began reading more about men who had the disease, I knew that I was not alone. One of my first exposures to prostate cancer had been through a man named Leo Madden—once a fixture at IBE.

From the beginning, Leo was one of those behind-the-scenes laborers in the vineyard so critical to building the foundation on which the IBE organization stands. Leo was the consummate team player. His job was whatever he had to do to make Expo better.

Leo's commitment to Expo was matched only by his love for God and family. The organization is greater today because he touched it.

Leo was the first man I knew who had prostate cancer. I was introduced to it through him long before the disease had anything to do with me, back in 1995—1998, from the time of his diagnosis until his death.

When doctors told Leo that his greatest prospects of prolonging life would require the surgical removal of his testicles, he refused. It would have required an intricate and traumatic procedure. Leo flatly rejected the idea. Even though he was in his early sixties, Leo felt that the operation would render him less than a man. Instead, he limited his options to hormone therapy.

As the months passed, Leo weakened. He became sick more often. His skin changed, becoming paler and drier. Two compassionate Expo staff members frequently visited him at home to give him a comforting rub down. But there would be no lasting comfort. Leo began losing weight and seemed to be fading fast. He was in a lot of pain. Through it all he remained a devoutly religious man, dedicated to his church and Christian faith. He played piano for the congregation as long as he could. Then Leo's notes were silenced on June 24, 1998.

Though I saw Leo change from a healthy, exuberant individual to a sickly, deteriorating man, I failed to take advantage of the opportunity to find out more about the "C" word. In my mind, Leo's tragedy had no relationship to my health because he was in his sixties and I was still in my forties. I attributed his cancer to old age. Those thoughts were born out of ignorance. By not walking with Leo through his ordeal, I lost a learning opportunity. I should have been more aware of the need to share Leo's travails mentally, physically and spiritually. In doing that, I would have not only been a greater comfort to him, I would have broadened my own understanding.

The lesson I learned too late for it to help me was simple enough: *Don't wait until you or someone you're close to is the patient before you bother to explore causes, prevention, treatments and facts about prostate cancer. Don't be reactive . . . be proactive.*

And don't let your new knowledge make you feel that you can start "playing doctor." The benefit of your research is that it allows you to ask good questions of your doctors, not to supplant or ignore their expertise. Doctors will respect your knowledge, and that makes it easier for you and your doctor to develop a good working relationship. You'll also be better able to make informed decisions about your treatments.

Now that I have a lot more time on my hands, I've learned to manage it more wisely—to use precious hours studying and compiling available resources about prostate cancer. Despite the fear you may occasionally feel by what you find, being well informed about prostate cancer, or any other cancer, is much better than being uninformed and ignorant.

Consider this: If you urge those men you love to stop smoking to avoid lung cancer, then shouldn't you also tell them to get checked for prostate? The likelihood is that prostate cancer will kill them before tobacco will—especially if they happen to be black.

The facts are that in 2001, the most commonly diagnosed cancers in African American men were:

- Prostate cancer: 37%
- Lung cancer: 15%
- Colon and rectal cancer: 9%

African American men need to stop, look and listen for the warning signs; they need to get tested. The first step is to realize that, according to the American Cancer Society, we are 47% more likely to get prostate cancer than white men and two or three times more likely to die from the disease. In fact, the National Cancer Institute has reported that black American males have the highest rate of prostate cancer in the world.

The American Cancer Society says the black male population in the U.S. suffers from prostate cancer at a population rate of 234.2 per 100,000 compared to only 144.6 per 100,000 whites. The death rate for African American males is 53.1 per 100,000 compared to 22.4 deaths per 100,000 male Caucasians. And the Cancer Society submits that the five-year survival rate for African American males is 92%—significantly below the 97% five-year survival rate for whites. This disease is taking out brothers at a rate that would cause a coast-to-coast uproar if everyone knew the truth.

It's encouraging that, finally, coalitions and proactive organizations, like the 100 Black Men, the Rainbow Coalition, Indiana Black Expo, black Greek-letter organizations, and dozens of other notable black church, civic and social entities with national audiences, are merging to fight against prostate cancer. Their unified involvement will have a dramatic impact and foster much-needed attention on the disease.

In this movement toward greater community understanding of prostate cancer, men can't do it alone. Women need to be proactive by insisting that the men in their lives prioritize health care and be tested. Whether we admit it or not, just about everything men do is for the opposite sex—from the time of boyhood to the grave. That puts women in a powerful position to help bring about awareness and early detection of the disease.

Most committed men strive to become good husbands and good fathers, good lovers and good friends to the women in their lives. Women garner strength to overcome obstacles by encouraging their partners. They look to them as a port in the storm of struggle. Men equally relish sharing achievements with their women. A good man strives to become a respectable provider, ample supporter, and caring partner.

If we accept the premise that men basically live for the women in their lives, then the power of women in this struggle can't be touted enough. Let the brothers know how manly it is to live, whether it means loss of some function or not. Discourage their "playing doctor" or waiting until a problem is severe before going to a doctor.

No public awareness campaign could be more persuasive than the gentle but firm insistence of women urging reluctant brothers to take the prostate-specific antigen (PSA) blood test and rectal examination for early detection.

Mothers tell your sons, wives tell your husbands, girlfriends tell your boyfriends, female relatives tell your male family members: These two simple tests for early detection of prostate cancer can make the difference between life or death.

Don't feel bad if you barely know what the prostate is or where it's located in the body. Many men with college degrees don't know. Most of us take the functions of our body for granted and only focus on otherwise obscure body parts when we, or the people we know, have problems with them.

Remember: Knowledge is power. It will be difficult for anyone to try to fight prostate cancer without being armed with knowledge. So let's look at the prostate itself and what it does.

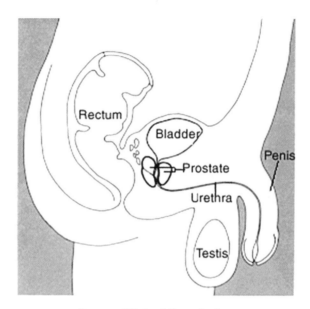

Courtesy of National Cancer Institute

The prostate is a small internal organ that can cause huge problems if something happens to it. The prostate is a sex gland located inside the lower abdomen at the base of the penis, just below the bladder. In its normal state, the prostate is about the size of a golf ball—an inch and a half in diameter. Its shape is that of an upside down pear.

The prostate wraps around the urethra, the tube that empties urine from the bladder through the penis. The prostate is connected to male reproductive organs. The two tubes that transport sperm from the testicles into the urethra and the two clusters of tiny sacs that contribute fluid to semen all drain into the prostate.

The prostate gland produces *prostatic fluid* that regulates the acidity of semen. Being high in alkaline, prostatic fluid protects sperm as it travels through the acid environment of the female reproductive tract.

The prostate also serves as a valve that allows sperm and urine to flow in the right direction out of the body through the urethra. The prostate acts as a pump. During an orgasm, prostate muscular tissues contract, forcing semen through the urethra. The bladder neck surrounding the urethra, near the base of the prostate, stops semen from flowing into the bladder during ejaculation.

Technically speaking, as valuable as it is, the prostate gland is not considered a vital organ. That is, men can survive without it, as they can survive without a gall bladder—though it makes life much more convenient to have these organs in good working condition.

A thin, fibrous membrane, sometimes called the *capsule* surrounds most of the prostate. If cancerous cells escape from the prostate gland beyond this outer layer, they can circulate to other parts of the body. From that point on, prostate cancer is more difficult to cure.

That's why early detection is so critical. Prostate cancer is slow in growing and is treatable. The sooner the cancer is found in the prostate, the easier it is to contain and control it. The chance of survival for those whose problem is caught in the first stage is extremely high.

The first test for prostate health you'll get is likely to be the digital rectal examination (DRE), which requires the physician to insert a gloved finger into the rectum. As silly as it may seem to some, especially women, this is one of the barriers to getting men tested. Heterosexual males are unaccustomed to anything penetrating their rectums. The apprehension seems almost laughable given its potential consequences. But it is real.

The prostate is divided into three zones. The largest is the peripheral zone, which contains about 70% of the prostate's glandular tissue. Most prostate cancer begins in this area. This is the only area a doctor can feel during a rectal exam and the area from which tissue is likely to be sampled for a biopsy.

The remaining prostate glandular tissue is found in the *central* and *transition zones.* The transition zone surrounds the urethra and is usually the smallest area of the three. Virtually all *benign prostatic hyperplasia (BPH)*—a non-cancerous enlargement of the prostate—is found in the transition zone.

Finally, the central zone is located at the base of the prostate nearest the bladder. Cancer rarely begins in that area.

The prostate is the size of a pea in little boys. Considerable growth occurs during adolescence, when the body produces large amounts of male hormones.

After a male becomes an adult, the prostate takes on its full size and shape. It does not normally grow any more until a man begins to age. The median age for men diagnosed with prostate cancer ranges from sixty to sixty-five years of age. But it's much younger for black men. That's why most doctors recommend that black men should begin to get tested for prostate cancer around the age of fifty. If there is a family history of the disease, it is recommended that testing begin as early as age forty.

When something triggers abnormal growth, prostate cancer can begin. The precise reason for this abnormal growth remains a medical mystery. Prostate cancer is influenced by heredity, environment and hormones, so each must be considered when attempting to determine one's level of risk for the disease.

Obesity may be a factor in the incidence of prostate cancer among African American males. The American Cancer Society released, in 2002, a study conducted by California researcher Christopher L. Ambling, M.D.—a urologist at the Naval

Medical Center in San Diego. Dr. Ambling examined medical data on 860 patients who underwent *prostatectomy* (surgical removal of the prostate gland) for prostate cancer at three military medical centers in the years 1992 through 1998.

Obese men made up 20% of all the men who had the procedure, while an additional 49% were classified as overweight. The study showed that obese men of all races were younger when diagnosed with prostate cancer and documented that these patients had cancer that was more advanced and aggressive. Obese men were more likely to have cancer that had already spread beyond the prostate.

Dr. Ambling found that twenty-seven percent of African American men in the study were obese, compared to 19% of white men and only 4% of Asian men. Though only 10% of the men in the study were black, African Americans were 17% of the obese group.

Dr. Ambling's study was one of the first to suggest that African American men are more likely to get prostate cancer— and to die from it—at least partly because that population is more obese.

Durado Brooks, M.D., MPH, director of prostate and colorectal cancer at the American Cancer Society, warned that Dr. Ambling's study raises interesting possibilities but requires further "sub group" study to be considered absolutely valid. However, Dr. Brooks affirmed that obesity raises the overall cancer risk as well as the risk of damage to the heart and blood vessels. He said a multi-dimensional approach to lowering cancer risks must include diet, exercise and screening. Dr. Brooks said that a man who maintains normal weight for his height and who has good diet and exercise habits, and who also is regularly screened for prostate cancer, is more likely to reduce the chance of prostate cancer.

There is more good news: The Radiological Society of Northwest America reported at their 88th annual meeting in Chicago in December, 2002 that African American men are just as likely as whites to be cured of prostate cancer when they are diagnosed early and treated with radioactive seeds implanted in the prostate.

Unfortunately, prostate cancer among African Americans is more frequently diagnosed after the cancer has *metastasized* or spread to regional or distant sites, within the body. While the incidence of men afflicted with prostate cancer is soaring, some reports indicate that the survival rate among those who detect the disease early is on the rise. But even given similar treatment at the same stage of disease as others, black men have a higher mortality rate.

The National Cancer Institute reported findings of a study conducted from 1983 to 1990. It found that the five-year survival rate for black American males was just over 65%. For white Americans, the survival rate for a comparable group during the same period was over 80%.

There is no single pill or medicine that works for every patient. Only professional caregivers are qualified to prescribe the best treatment for an individual. It's important that patients do their homework and offer input into the decision.

It is important to be honest about your reaction to a medication or treatment once it begins and to keep your health care team informed if you have a bad reaction. Cooperation and truthfulness between you, your doctor, and your other health care providers is essential to your successful treatment.

Finally, the ultimate key—in conjunction with the medications your doctor prescribes—is prayer. For any real chance of recovery the patient must be willing to put up a spirited, good fight.

So work with your doctor, know your medications. Understand your treatments. Do your research. Ask questions. Pray. It's a powerful combination!

In my case, the medications on page 78 have been prescribed at one time or another during my treatment.

CANCER

- Lupron injection
- Zometa
- Casodex
- Coumadin

CHEMOTHERAPY

- Emcyt
- Decadron
- Taxotere
- Dexamethasone

HIGH BLOOD PRESSURE

- Prinivil
- Demadex
- Lisinopril
- Norvasc
- Toprol XL

PAIN

- Oxycontin
- Analgesic patches
- Hodrocodene

NAUSEA

- Prochlorperazine

ARTHRITIS

- Cellebrex
- Vioxx

CONSTIPATION AND FLATULENCE

- Senekot
- Tums
- Citricell
- Gas-X

CHAPTER SIX

WHISPERS AND SHOUTS

From the moment of my diagnosis, God began using me as an instrument for change. Once I managed to get past my own paralyzing first reaction, feeling like I had just entered the twilight zone, it was as though a road map had been thrust in my face to guide me through my unexpected journey. However unknown the course, it was comforting to know that God would direct my path.

The first step was to proclaim that "yes," I do have incurable prostate cancer but "no," I'm not planning on going anywhere soon. How could I be so certain? Simple, I had a little talk with Jesus.

The second step was to use my visibility to inform black men and those who love them how important it is to take prostate cancer seriously. By the spring of 2003, my story had been told on radio and television public service announcements, through public speaking appearances, in newspaper articles and columns, and through my participation in local support groups.

The results have been heartening. Eastern Star Church—one of the largest and most prestigious congregations in Indianapolis—

hosted a Men's Forum and Health Fair in my honor that included prostate cancer (PSA), cholesterol, high blood pressure and stroke screening. The Health Fair also included panel discussions geared toward education and prevention.

Just as important, rather than being the act of a single interest, the event actually represented a coalition of Eastern Star Church with the Marion County Health Department, Indiana Black Expo, Kappa Alpha Psi Fraternity, Little Red Door and other local business and civic partners.

The screening sessions started shortly after 9 o'clock on a Saturday morning. By the time the fair was scheduled to close four hours later, the lines of African American men waiting to be screened still stretched around the length of the gymnasium and out the door, Throughout the day, the longest line was the one for prostate cancer screening.

This event proved two things: First, that a local leader's health disclosure could enhance public awareness of a health issue. Second, that the news and example of my own delay seemed to have an immediate effect on men wary of making the same error.

If the massive response to free screening was indeed a reaction to my disclosure, it provides yet another reason for me to celebrate the way in which the Lord guides me, and strengthens my will to continue this crucial mission.

On the human side, going public raises the question of how others will react. I hoped to avoid those piteous *whispers* from people who tend to fear for the worst. At the same time, I didn't look forward to encountering the over-exuberant *shouts* from folks trying to camouflage their sadness or confusion or ambivalence with a guarantee of my immediate and complete recovery.

I know there is only one who holds my future, and truly believe that God has already worked it out according to his perfect will. I have already claimed the victory.

The agitation of the whispers is that they tend to over-dramatize my predicament. The equally annoying shouts seem to dismiss or trivialize the very real and present pain endured by patients. Sometimes even those who have the best intentions can do or say things that contribute to, rather than assuage, the suffering. A pat on the back isn't necessarily helpful if the person's ailment happens to be a sore back.

This, however, does not lessen the appreciation I have for all those who care enough to express themselves. I'm only suggesting that when it comes to reactions, most ill patients who have been labeled "terminal " probably prefer folks to be somewhere between the overly cautious, too-polite whispers and the over compensating, far too zealous shouts.

Just be natural. Ideal are those friends and strangers who react with a combination of heartfelt empathy rising above a whisper, tempered with firm confidence in the power of recovery through prayer. You sense what's in the heart and that's what matters most.

Some of the most inspirational responses to my plight have come from a special blend of family members, high-profile businessmen, elected officials and community stalwarts in Indianapolis, along with strangers and friends from around the country who offer sincere prayer.

For example, Indianapolis business magnate William G. Mays—owner of one of the most successful black-owned enterprises in the U.S., Mays Chemicals, is also a close friend and chairman of the Circle City Classic Board. Mays volunteered his financial resources to assist me in getting the best medical treatments available, and to help me with any of my daily needs. His gesture was moving beyond words, and brought tears to my eyes.

Indianapolis Colts team owner Bill Irsay is an individual with whom I have enjoyed a long association and close friendship. When he learned of my diagnosis of prostate cancer, he offered to provide his private jet to fly me anywhere in the country, or the world, that I needed to go while engaged in this fight to survive.

These demonstrations of genuine concern uplift me immensely. They also reassure me that there is a good reason God put such beautiful people in my life, and me in theirs. Perhaps these friends see something in my spirit that assures them I would do the same for them if our roles were reversed. These friends affirm my lifelong ambition to make an impact through service.

Reactions to my disclosure include a flurry of communications with people who also have prostate cancer. Many say that but for my example they would have kept the situation to themselves.

One personal friend who served as a mentor to me thirty years ago stopped me in the hallway of the Indianapolis convention center and told me that he was in his third year after being diagnosed with prostate cancer. He said he was encouraged by my forthcoming attitude. He said that it influenced him to reveal his condition to close friends and fellow professionals.

Another revelation came during a casual conversation with Dusty Baker, the manager of the Chicago Cubs, who in 2002 guided the San Francisco Giants to the National League championship. Speaking of the challenge that I was confronting, Baker confessed that he too was coping with prostate cancer.

The example of how he has gone on with his life and continued to grow professionally has helped me understand that life does go on, and great things can be accomplished. Obviously, Dusty Baker was diagnosed at an earlier stage than I was, which just emphasized yet again that it is much more than rhetoric to declare that black men should aggressively monitor their own health.

Both candid conversations materialized only because I was willing to go public with my battle. And both confirmed my feelings about the tremendous positive ripple effect of black men telling the people in their lives about their illnesses. Being silent won't make the pain any easier to endure. Indeed, speaking out has lightened my load because I now can and do share my feelings openly with others. Why suffer alone?

Many say that they hesitate to make their illness known to individuals outside their immediate families because they fear the reaction of others. Sadly, these people opt to keep their illness private and safe from any unwanted scrutiny. Many fear, or are ashamed of, the stigma attached to impotence.

My response is that none of us has anything at all to be ashamed of. Impotence can diminish one's spirit, and wreak havoc on our self-esteem. But that too can be overcome, if and when you truly face it.

One of my most fervent hopes is that by speaking out, I will encourage more men who already have prostate cancer to re-examine their silence. We need to learn from each other and garner strength from one another's experiences.

People of all races and economic levels have shown much love, offered their assistance, blessed my family, my circumstances, and me with their prayers. Those gifts have been a powerful resource in my struggle to defeat the odds. I humbly and graciously receive them as a privilege and an honor.

Fielding the mixed bag of reactions is sometimes the hard part. No matter what you expect, you can never be quite sure how people will react to your ordeal. Some show more shock than you did when doctors gave you the news. For others, hugs and tears speak for them.

Some told me about people that they knew of or read about somewhere who had prostate cancer and pulled through. It's so easy for someone to almost nonchalantly say that they know I'm going to be fine soon because they read somewhere about a man—or they have a relative or a friend or a neighbor –who survived prostate cancer with little difficulty.

Well I can tell you firsthand, so far there has been nothing easy about this journey. But I remain encouraged as I meditate daily on the words of Helen Keller, "Character cannot be developed in ease and quiet. Only through experience of trial and suffering can the soul be strengthened, ambition inspired, and success achieved."

My relationship with the Lord remains unshaken.

What I have discovered is that far too many men remain unaware of the unforgiving nature of waiting too late. To compare the outcome of those diagnosed in the first two stages of prostate cancer with the outcome of people whose illness is unveiled in the final stage is like comparing the effects of drinking water to those of drinking alcohol.

I've also encountered people who are just unable to find the right expression. Rather than shout, whisper or offer any course in between, they change the subject and look for the first chance to escape. I understand.

But I have less tolerance for those whose approach is either rude or insensitive. The classic non-thinker responds with the morose, "Well, nobody lives forever," or "We all have to go sometime," or coldly suggests that I focus only on getting my affairs in order. Having cancer doesn't make you "jerk proof." The bottom line is that when a prostate cancer patient decides to spread the word, he should be prepared for anything and everything in terms of responses.

While the vast majority of people I've encountered applaud my candor, one surprising reaction came from a source close to my heart, my youngest son, Charles II. His point blank question: "Why did you have to go and tell everybody?"

It caught me completely off guard. No one else inquired, even if they wondered. And certainly no one else had expressed to me that they thought my openness was inappropriate. But my son, who holds a main line to my heart, and is a major part of my life, challenged the wisdom of both my decision and my actions. As the conversation between us progressed, it became apparent that part of his concern was the awkwardness of fielding questions from high school classmates who read of my illness in the *Indianapolis Star*. Later we would resolve his concerns about my disclosure, but for now, I was proud that he felt comfortable enough to talk openly to me about his feelings. In his own way, he was talking freely and disclosing his own thoughts and emotions.

The Lord works in mysterious ways. Prayers, telephone calls, letters and emails that flow in regularly from compassionate individuals across the country offer me continuous encouragement. But deeper reactions to my illness have transformed what could have been for me a period of exasperating gloom to a time of exhilarating promise.

Two reactions have stirred me most: The first, of course, is the offer of prayer from so many. I believe in my heart that God answers. And black men who don't happen to be in the public light are just as entitled to respect and prayer as those who are. Our titles and accomplishments are not as important as the commitment of our hearts. And it doesn't take tens of thousands of people to make your prayer link powerful. All it takes is one sincere heart and the connection is made straight to the One who counts most.

The second reaction I've found compelling is when someone shares with me that my example encouraged him to get a prostate cancer exam. In the end, what matters most is that black men might live. I am already claiming my victory by faith. Thus, my mission is that other black men might acquire my knowledge—and more—and use it to respond to this illness, and others, in a way that promotes long and healthy lives.

Whenever anyone reacts to my situation with doubt or sorrow, I won't have it. I reject those deceptive notions out of the strength of my conviction and emphasize that my challenge lies in reaching far beyond one man. My book is about drawing attention to the struggle of anonymous black men coast to coast who are already battling prostate cancer. And it's about eliminating the dubious distinction that African American men are hardest hit by the illness.

During a particularly down day in February, 2003, one poignant piece of poetry sent to me sums up my sentiments well. The poem, by Syble Simmons, is entitled, *"Life's Not All About Me."*

Though my troubles and my worries
Are sometimes all that I can see

Still I always must remember
Life's not all about me.
Other souls are also hurting
And I know that it's God's plan
To reach out to help another
To extend to them my hand.
With this purpose as my focus
To be a comfort to a friend
All my troubles and my worries
Seem to fade out in the end.
It is one of God's true lessons
How my walk is meant to be
True happiness I find when
Life is not only about me.

Perhaps the most valuable help I've received comes from the elite community of cancer survivors. Whether it is colon, breast, lung or any other form of the disease, there is a kindred aura and spirit among those who pull through. One such individual is Thomas W. Dortch Jr., chairman of the board of The100 Black Men of America. Dortch won his battle with intestinal cancer. When he heard about my diagnosis, he talked to me about his personal experience with the disease and how his organization was helping to spread the word about prostate screening. Here are his answers to my questions:

Q: Tell us about your experience with cancer.
Everyone wonders from time to time how he or she will depart this world. Because my father died of a massive heart attack and earlier battled diabetes, becoming a victim of cancer was the last

thing on my mind. When I first began having abdominal pains, I thought it might be an ulcer. Because of my discipline, I sought medical support to determine my problem. Several tests produced no results but I refused to give up. Finally after exploratory surgery and a CAT scan, a mass in my small intestines was revealed. Doctors at first thought it was a cyst. When the tests came back though, they showed that I had a rare form of intestinal cancer with a 92 percent mortality. Because of my faith and two young children at the time, I was determined to overcome the odds. Because of a positive attitude, strong family support, expert medical care and a resounding faith in God, I was blessed to survive. That happened in 1989.

Q: What was most difficult about your struggle?
The first part is the unknown. Cancer is a dreaded disease that everybody fears. It is taboo to discuss it in the black community, so many of us have no opportunities to talk to other survivors, to understand their struggles and to benefit from their counsel on how best to combat disease from a mental standpoint.

The other difficulty was finding myself, an exceptionally active and busy thirty-eight-year-old man, suddenly confined to my home or the hospital for long periods of time after surgery and chemotherapy.

Q: Where did you find greatest comfort?
My family. My children. My vision for what I wanted to do to help rebuild my community and to help young people succeed.

Q: How has intestinal cancer most changed your life?

I find myself seeking ways to avoid stress. Since childhood, everyone talked about trying to eat the right foods to avoid cancer. Nobody ever talked about how important it is to avoid stress. I found out too late how stress breaks down the body's immune systems, making it more susceptible to disease. I also find myself walking and getting more exercise. Finally, I get regular checkups with my oncologist, urologist and general practitioner.

Q: Why is more said today about prostate cancer than before?

Prostate cancer has been around for centuries. Any man who lives long enough will likely develop it. Sometimes it may have no impact. Because African American males are so much more likely to get prostate cancer, 100 Black Men has formed the "Prostate Cancer Coalition." More doctors are talking about the disease than before. Finally, more people are being urged to have a regular prostate exam with their annual physical.

While the disease has always been around, it has drawn more attention because of many well-known individuals who have battled it. The list includes Michael Milken, Andrew Young, Dusty Baker, and Minister Louis Farrakhan.

Q: What should black men do first?

African American men should change their diets—adding more protein and reducing fat. They should also exercise more and stress themselves out less. Consumption of alcohol should be lessened. Finally, check-ups on a regular basis are essential.

Q: What are your thoughts on alternative drugs and treatments?
There are documented success stories of people who fought prostate cancer with herbs and the holistic approach. There have also been successes with more conventional treatment. My only advice is for individuals to research and educate themselves and seek the guidance of professionals before making a decision.

Q: Can you discuss preferred treatment options for prostate cancer?
That is a matter left to each individual patient and the medical team.

Q: How can we better fight prostate cancer on the national level?
The one thing that I adamantly believe is that there must be more extensive commitment to research on prostate cancer. We can spend billions to go to war, so there must be money for prostate cancer and other diseases that afflict American citizens. There needs to be a better campaign for public awareness.

Q: What can women do in this struggle for early detection?
Spouses, daughters and the entire female community have a tremendous role to play. They have the power of influence. It is important for them to encourage, and if necessary 'nag,' stubborn black men to get exams and change bad habits.

Q: Should black celebrities and churches do more?
Everybody has to play a role. The hip-hop community has the ears of so many. If they place healthcare at the top of their

agenda, it would push young people to be more conscientious. The younger generation can also influence corporations, the music industry, athletes and stars of screen and television to get involved. The church is valuable because it has a captive audience. Preachers need to preach the message of healthcare more often. The bottom line is that everybody needs to do more.

Q: Why are black men so nonchalant about their health?
It's partly our culture. Black men are so macho they don't think that they can get sick. If they do, they feel they can just get over it if they weather the storm. It's amazing how many people casually say; "I don't know what's bothering me." In fact, they could be dying and could be saved. For some it's economic. They don't consider medical care a priority. For others, it's just simple ignorance. If we don't wake up, we are going to continue to die when we could be treated and survive. With better nutrition, exercise and check-ups, we can be a healthier people, live longer and live better.

Q: What is The 100 Black Men of America doing about prostate cancer prevention and awareness?
Our organization dates back to 1994. We have adopted a plan called "Four for the Future" and everything that we do falls into one of these categories. The four categories are education, mentoring, wellness and economic development. We are conducting prostate screenings throughout the country and internationally where we have chapters. We are also partnering with the Morehouse School of Medicine, working with Drs. James Gavin, Lewis Sullivan and David Satcher to dedicate more research to health care delivery and education throughout the African American and minority communities.

CHAPTER SEVEN

WHY US?

WHY PROSTATE CANCER HURTS
BLACK MEN MORE

I n the beginning, I asked, "Why me?" As time passed and my knowledge of prostate cancer grew, the question became "Why us?"

Of all the men on earth, why are black Americans more susceptible to prostate cancer and more severely ravaged by it? Is it genetics? Is it lifestyle? Is it diet? Is it health care? Is it economics? Is it ignorance?

"Why us?"

As we've seen, the facts depict an American enigma. Not only do black men have a higher incidence of prostate cancer, but we also have a lower rate of survival.

Prostate cancer among black men is more frequently diagnosed after the cancer has spread to regional or distant sites within the body. This is one reason black men in the U.S. have the highest death rate from the disease. The chance for surviving five years or longer after diagnosis is 81% for whites but only 66% for Blacks. These facts come from the National Cancer

Institute report, "Prostate Cancer and the African American Male," published in 1998. They are confirmed in virtually every other study that followed.

The cavalier attitude with which I handled my own warning signs wasn't too different from the way many black men handle personal health. From Oakland to Baltimore, from Minneapolis-St. Paul to Birmingham, while black men are diverse in thoughts and interest, we definitely share some cultural and social bonds that inextricably tie us together.

Many black men feel the need to constantly reassert their manhood. From personal life to the work place, no other racial or ethnic group has had to endure denigrating pangs of racism in the U.S. to the extent of the black man.

So do we sometimes act too tough or "macho" to camouflage our pain and vulnerability? Definitely. Are we sometimes too stubborn to heed advice because of our sense of assertiveness and self-determination? Frequently. Are there times when we ignore the best advice, and even our own better judgment, in favor of instincts and chance? Absolutely. Black men love to gamble against the odds because the odds are so often against us.

Even with these factors as part of the equation, the answer to the question still isn't clear. There are whites and men of all ethnicities who demonstrate the same characteristics. Why then is the price that the black man has to pay so high? Why do we have such a comparatively smaller margin of error?

There are few diseases that readily come to mind that don't hit people of color harder. The agonizing question remains. Why?

Some of the disparity, at least among prostate cancer victims according to many medical experts, is attributable to our high-fat diet. The next chapter will offer specific ways in which unhealthy eating can be turned around. Though diet is an aggravating factor, it's not the only link between blacks and prostate cancer.

The poverty rate among black Americans is twice that of whites and there's a correlation between income status and the ability to obtain higher quality health care and treatment. That's not debatable. Further, the cost of medication for minor illnesses is high. It skyrockets when you get to diseases like cancer. The National Cancer Institute (NCI) report confirms that nearly 62% of patients at clinics that serve predominately African Americans suffer more pain partially because they did not receive adequate pain medication.

Complicating the problem is the inability of many African American men to afford testing and treatment. Without adequate insurance, the cost of such a serious illness is enough to make you sick. The prostate exam can cost about $70. A follow-up biopsy will cost approximately $1,500 and if cancer is detected, the first year of treatment alone can top $30,000. Unemployment is twice as high for blacks (about 9%) as for whites (just over 4%). Black married couples are far less likely than white couples to have an annual income of $50,000 or more. And the poverty rate in black America is about 26% compared to approximately 8% among whites in the U.S.

Poverty is a concern, but not an absolute.

The Rev. Jesse Jackson illustrates the point. The former presidential candidate noted that much-needed national health insurance plans will be of little or no consequence if the lack of healthier lifestyles and extensive research is not addressed in the ongoing attempt to understand the question of why African American's suffer most severely when it comes to prostate cancer.

Insurance won't substitute for preventive measures, says Rev. Jackson, adding:

Insurance is not a health system, it's a health care system. The determination to get annual check ups and to honor the doctor's advice about food and diet and exercise and medicine are critical. Insurance does not inspire one to good health care habits. Insurance is simply a health care finance system.

I've gone to many union meetings to speak where people are concerned about health insurance coverage. The irony is that sometimes the smoke would be so thick that you almost had to wear an oxygen mask. And yet they are calling for a comprehensive health care system as they cough through the smoke. It doesn't make sense.

Insurance or the ability to pay can't save you from cancer. It can only help you pay for treatment. It's hypocrisy for someone to be coughing from their cigarette in one breath and arguing for better health care insurance in the next. You can't violate all the dietary laws, refuse to get screening, then blame your illness on the lack of proper insurance."

Rev. Jackson is right. The money factor is a serious concern, but not an absolute solution. Insurance is a red herring for too many African American men, diverting focus from more finite variables.

Most of us knew before anyone studied the facts that finances prevent many people of lower income from seeking and receiving the type of medical attention they need. Is the HIV-positive individual on the street likely to receive the same treatment and options as Magic Johnson? Of course not. But the question of 'why?' can't be answered simply through studying economics.

How do we account for the high incidence of prostate cancer among African American men who have money, a family doctor, healthier diets than most, a good education and a regular exercise regimen? And how do we begin to understand reports that show us that even when a black man and white man are diagnosed with the same stage of cancer, the African American patient will often not fare as well in the end?

Why us?

In truth, it's a question that has puzzled medical researchers for years. In the political correctness of America, it can be a touchy subject to suggest that the difference in the physical make-up of blacks and whites is more than skin deep. But at least two major studies hypothesize that biological differences between blacks and whites may play a greater role in health issues than previously believed.

In December, 2000, researchers at Harvard University published results of a ten-year study that tracked the incidence of prostate cancer in a group of more than 45,000 black and white male doctors, pharmacists, optometrists and other health professionals. In the study, African Americans were nearly twice as likely to develop prostate cancer.

The black and white men in this study had similar incomes, educational backgrounds, eating habits and access to quality healthcare. Interpreters of the study concluded that lifestyle probably had little or no influence on the risk of prostate cancer within this controlled group of men.

But there was a scientific distinction made between black and white men who participated in the study.

Proteins called androgen receptors on prostate cells were more likely to have a slight alteration in African American men.

Because these androgen receptors bind with hormones, such as testosterone, to promote the growth of prostate cancer, the Harvard study concluded that this variation in androgen receptors among blacks could explain a small portion of the higher prostate cancer rate.

In another study, researchers at Louisiana State University noticed that black men tend to have far more blood vessels than whites. Blacks were found to have genes that speed production of a protein known as TIMP-1 at about twenty times the rate of whites. TIMP-1 accelerates the growth of blood vessels. Consequently, those additional vessels around tumors spread malignant cells throughout the body much more quickly, according to LSU researchers.

Why is this protein so high in black men? Scientists at the LSU Health Sciences Center aren't sure, but one theory is that the production of TIMP-1 may be triggered by cholesterol in the diet. Men whose diets are rich in saturated fat, which raises cholesterol, are more likely to develop prostate cancer.

Such diets are usually more common among black men than white.

Dr. Charles J. McDonald of the American Cancer Society is one of the most significant medical authorities in the U.S. trying to find out why black men are so much more likely to get prostate cancer than whites and why black men are two to three times more likely than white men to die from it.

Like many medical professionals and scientists concerned with this mystery, Dr. McDonald isn't just talking about black men and prostate cancer—he's doing something about it. He has developed a blueprint that outlines action in four categories—

research, education, patient/family support and public policy measures. The five challenges he outlines are as follows:

1. Increase research, especially in relation to African American men, specifically examining causes, risk factors, preventive measures, and new effective treatments for prostate cancer.

2. Involve African American men in research design, in the implementation of clinical research, in the development of educational initiatives, and as patient participants in clinical research trials.

3. Develop effective educational programs about prostate cancer, not only for the public but also for health care professionals, especially primary care physicians.

4. Strengthen the capacity of grassroots organizations, particularly in the African American community, to effectively engage in advocacy and in educational and patient support initiatives.

5. Develop more community-based educational support and guidance programs for patients with prostate cancer and their families to help guide them through a frightening and confusing process.

Indiana Black Expo, Inc. joins in that call to action. The one thing that has to take place in order to definitely uncover answers to "Why us?" is the creation of strong coalitions among health care agencies, organizations, churches, corporations, the government, educators and concerned citizens across the nation. Those committed to America's future must make prostate cancer a national priority. Too often in the past, problems that predominantly effected blacks were ignored, addressed with no particular urgency, or put on a back burner. We can't let this happen with prostate cancer.

Understanding evolves from scientific research and theory. Still, the fact remains that no one knows exactly why blacks are hit hardest by prostate cancer, and the answer may not be revealed during our lifetimes. But whenever it happens, knowledge of the "why" will still just be one step in fighting the illness. Even when scientists finally pinpoint the exact causes for the disparity of prostate cancer rates between blacks and whites, they will have to determine what can be done with that information to even the playing field. They will need a cure equally effective for all.

It's heartening to know that impressive research continues in the quest for answers. But it's not enough. We can—and we must—help change happen. All of us have the power to petition those we elect to office to do more. From municipal and state government, to federal and world leadership, there is a need for more pressure to make research on blacks and prostate cancer a higher priority. If blacks aren't politically active, it won't happen. We have to make our voices heard individually and collectively.

Eventually, all the answers will be known. It may even happen sooner than we think. At this point, most importantly, is the question of what should we do in the interim? While we're waiting for the conclusive revelation of causes and effects, all we have to work with is what we know now about prostate cancer. We can't allow ourselves to remain dormant until the illness is eradicated.

Whatever the reason for the disproportionate rates of prostate cancer, two factors present clear obstacles to overcoming this tragedy.

The first is ignorance. The second is fear. Like me, many black men aren't deprived of information. It's available everywhere. Many of us, however, make a conscious choice to shy away from discussion of it because the subject is so frightening. Yet there's no shame in fear. We're all human. The shame is in allowing those apprehensions to rule our logic and common sense—to taint our judgment, to keep us from acting in our own best interests. Ignoring prostate cancer won't make it go away.

Get tested, black men. Instead of dwelling on selfish emotions we must think beyond them—about that child, that grandchild, that "soul mate" who may be deprived of your loving company as a result of pure negligence. Just think of the wonderful things in their lives that you may miss. Think of how they have come to depend on you, are inspired by you and are there for you whenever needed. Sometimes thinking beyond our selves is the jolt we need to push us into the unknown.

At Howard University Cancer Center, researcher Flora Ukoli pursues the theory that diet accounts for a significant portion of prostate cancer among black men. The primary obstacle in her research, Ukoli said, was the difficulty in finding enough men willing to participate in the study.

Imagine. Howard is located in predominantly black Washington, D.C. And prostate cancer is far more prevalent in blacks. Yet, that important research was stalled by the lack of willing participants. It's ironic and sad. By our reluctance to get involved in the research for prevention and cure, we hamper the very research that could provide answers to the question of 'why us?'

The time for soft-selling the need for African American men to be more responsive to their health needs has long passed. It's up to us, now. Nobody will save black men from themselves. Sensible, passionate appeals to get men screened are often lost on those who prefer Russian roulette to wrestling free from the manacles of fear.

Maybe screening should be a requirement for employment. The outcome of undetected prostate cancer can be far worse than that of drug addiction, and yet employers don't hesitate to screen for that. Maybe the Bureau of Motor Vehicles of each state across America should require license renewal to include rectal and PSA examinations for black male motorists over forty.

I'm being facetious, of course. Sometimes I have to laugh to keep from crying. But prostate cancer is no joke. And no matter what researchers come up with in laboratories, if the individual African American man isn't willing to take some responsibility for his fate, no experiment to find the answers to 'why us' will make a difference.

That reality can't be expressed strongly or often enough. It's painfully simple. Early screening means earlier diagnosis. Earlier diagnosis expands options for treatment. The more doctors, urologists and oncologists are in a position to do for you, the better the chance of eventually resuming your normal life. You don't have to be a scientist to appreciate that formula.

Chapter Eight

NO STONE UNTURNED

DIET, EXERCISE AND HERBS

To go from being virtually drug-free to a regimen of eleven different pills, each one taken one to three times a day, is a considerable adjustment. Now it's a way of life for me. But medicine, surgery and treatments are only part of the picture when it comes to the care and maintenance of one with cancer.

Along with the most advanced procedures, the most innovative therapy, and the latest drugs, a key factor relating to prostate cancer, as mentioned in earlier chapters, is diet. It's true that we are what we eat. So let's examine ways to improve our diets to reduce the risk of prostate cancer.

Remember, I'm not a nutrition expert. The information that follows, though, is compiled from people who are. So before making any dramatic dietary change don't take my word for it; be sure to check with your doctor.

Just as you don't fight an enemy with a single weapon, it's important that we leave no stone unturned in the search for the prevention, treatment and cure of prostate cancer.

If I knew before my illness what I know now, I would have made the sacrifice of what tastes good for what was in good taste years ago. But I was like everyone else. Though I read newspaper and magazine articles, watched television news and documentaries, and even personally knew individuals who suffered prostate cancer, I was never inspired to make real permanent changes until I became the patient. Diet is often a force of habit. The transformation from living to eat to eating to live has made me much more conscientious about:

- drinking more water (even though I never acquired a taste for it).
- eating foods with less fat
- eating more fruit and vegetables
- replacing dairy products and meats with soy products and fish

Yes, we are all occasionally guilty of the "it won't happen to me" syndrome. It doesn't make us bad people—just naïve people. Likewise, throughout our lives, most of us overcome one physical challenge after another without surrendering to our self-destructive behaviors. For example, those who chronically overeat may frequently rely on antacids for temporary relief and the seamstress who can let out the seams of our clothing another couple of inches to keep us in clothes that fit. In short, it's often easier for people to revert to a quick fix, to cheat on themselves just a little, than to attempt life-altering changes.

But if we decided to live healthier before we became sick, think of the suffering we might avoid in the future.

Diet influences the probability and effects of cancer. That's not medical theory, it is scientific fact. Yet even armed with that knowledge, many otherwise intelligent people ignore the potential good or harm of the food we choose, just as did I.

The biggest lie is that 'if it's good to you . . . it's good for you.' I'm a witness. When you commit to a diet of so-called "health food," you may sacrifice some of the taste to which you may be accustomed. But take it from a man who always loved a hearty meal, when it comes to life and death, the most savory thing is to stay alive and live well. And the truth is, many of the foods that are good for you also taste great too!

To stay healthy, you'll absolutely have to develop the strength to kick that handy "drive through" habit. Few items at the fast food restaurants would make the cancer prevention menu. To benefit from healthier eating, diet can't be approached like a fad that you hit for a few weeks then quit. If you don't plan to make a lasting change, you're fooling yourself.

Too seldom did I push myself away from the table. I spent most of my life overweight. At one point, I tipped the scales at 383 pounds. Because of my position and personality, weight was not a factor in my professional or personal life. The people that I worked or socialized with saw the bulging pounds but they didn't see them. I was just "Rev" or Charles.

But when I stepped out of that friendly environment, life was sometimes less kind. Those who suffer obesity know the embarrassment of trying to squeeze into a regular seat on an airplane or at the theater. At the heaviest point of my life, tipping the scales at almost 400 pounds, I had to pay for two airline tickets because of my girth. At that dismal point, when I went to the hospital, doctors had to weigh me on a truck scale.

That risky lifestyle actually posed a double threat. Not only were the food choices unhealthy, but the resulting obesity also contributed to the risk of prostate cancer, not to mention high blood pressure, diabetes, and other illnesses.

Dr. Steven Clinton of the Dana-Farber Cancer Institute wrote a publication entitled, *Prostate Cancer: A Multidisciplinary Guide*, in which he says that based on scientific evidence the following eight-point program significantly lowers the risk of prostate cancer:

1. Maintain a healthy body weight and exercise regularly.

2. Eat foods low in total fat and cholesterol. Select foods and ingredients with unsaturated fats instead of saturated fats.

3. Eat at least five servings of fresh fruit and vegetables per day. Some studies show that tomatoes, in particular, lower the risk of prostate cancer.

4. Aim to make carbohydrates 55-60 percent of your daily diet calories, especially complex carbohydrates such as those found in breads, whole grain cereals, pasta and rice.

5. Eat meats in moderation. This will limit your intake of high amounts of fat and cholesterol, both of which are found in most meat products.

6. Eat sugar and salt in moderation (though there has been no link of these substances to prostate cancer).

7. Drink alcohol in moderation, if at all.

8. Consume a variety of healthy foods for a balanced diet.

Among the best anti-cancer foods are:

- broccoli
- cabbage
- brussels sprouts
- carrots

- cauliflower
- kale
- peppers
- radishes
- squash
- eggplant
- green beans
- red onions
- soy beans
- sweet potatoes/yams

Some of the best cancer fighting fruits are:

- apricots
- blueberries
- grapefruit
- oranges
- peaches
- strawberries
- lemons
- mangoes
- grapes
- papayas
- persimmons
- tangerines

Our daily diets should contain no more than 20% fat. If we eat 2,500 calories, for example, fat should account for no more than 500 of those calories. That comes out to about 55 grams of fat per day. Even then, we have to consume 'the right fat.' Some fat, such as unsaturated fats found in plant foods, and vegetable oils high in monounsaturated fats, such as olive oil and canola oil, don't contribute to cancer. Studies show that men who eat less animal fat and more vegetable fat are less likely to have prostate cancer.

The more harmful fats are saturated fats such as palm, palm kernel, coconut and cottonseed oils and hydrogenated fats that have been chemically changed. Nearly all packaged foods, such as potato chips, contain hydrogenated fats, which help give them a longer shelf life.

How easy is it to eat healthily? Very.

- Have a bowl of high fiber bran cereal for breakfast.
- Eat beans regularly.
- Make your main meal a huge salad—with no more than a tablespoon of vegetable oil as dressing. Make it with dark green leafy spinach and other dark green leafy vegetables (instead of iceberg lettuce, which is nutritionally useless). Throw in broccoli, red pepper, beans of all kinds, garlic.

These dietary choices are simple and easy to implement. More dietary recommendations are available from "PSA Rising," a magazine that focuses exclusively on prostate cancer (psa-rising.com). Also in that Internet publication are a variety of results from cutting edge studies on prostate cancer. A few of the recent studies mentioned in "PSA Rising" include:,

- A Duke University Medical Center study in which a diet that contains flaxseed is identified as a possible factor in not only warding off prostate cancer in mice but also for reducing the size, aggressiveness, and severity of their tumors.
- A report that consumption of fatty fish such as salmon, sardine, herring and mackerel may reduce the risk of prostate cancer by one third.
- A report that men with prostate cancer might eat soy products in place of meat, poultry, cow's milk, cheese and other animal-based foods. (Keep in mind that the Food and Drug Administration discourages treating soy as a medicine or drug.)

- A study conducted at Oregon State University in April, 2000 which revealed that white tea, known mostly to tea connoisseurs, may have the strongest potential of all teas for fighting cancer. Tea, which is high in antioxidants, is helpful in warding off many forms of cancer.
- According to an Australian study, eating three times the recommended daily intake of folate and vitamin B12 may lower the risk factors of cancer by protecting your DNA. Folate-rich foods include leafy green vegetables and whole grains. Vitamin B12 is found in meat, chicken, fish, liver and kidneys or in supplement form. Two compounds from edible plants—one from grains and the other from fruits and vegetables—suppress the growth of three kinds of human cancer cells in the laboratory, according to researchers at the University of Wisconsin-Madison. Their findings support the theory that diets rich in plants are beneficial in fighting prostate cancer.

Other studies show further possible advances:

- Citrus limonoides, found in orange peel and other citrus rinds, could have significant health benefits, scientists reported at a meeting of the American Chemical Society in April, 1999. The active compound may have anti-cancer effects. Citrus limonoids are present in commercial orange juice at about the same level as vitamin C.
- Lifelong intake of potassium, magnesium, fruits and vegetables positively affect bone strength as we age. That is

important in connection with prostate cancer because men who have it may be afflicted with two different bone conditions—osteoporosis (or bone loss) and the spread of cancer to the bones (which has occurred in my case).

Even to a lay person it sounds logical that if foods from plants are most helpful in preventing cancer, herbs extracted from plants should also have some power to fight cancer.

That logic led me to consult an Amish practitioner.

I had heard over the last couple of years about people going to Amish practitioners and getting herbs that cured cancer. I've always been a little skeptical. If something is not FDA (Federal Drug Administration) approved, it's worrisome to me. I had so many people call me and write me about cancer-curing products that I had to be sure in my mind that this wasn't just another unconventional, untested scheme.

Then I reflected on my mother's bout with breast cancer. She used various herbs and claimed that they helped the healing process. People who are sick want very badly to be well. My mother is a very spiritual person. When I saw her using herbs, I remained cynical, taking a 'we'll see' attitude. Well, my mother turned seventy-six in 2003 and looks even younger now than before her bout with breast cancer.

I told my radiation oncologist about my plans to visit the Amish practitioner. She said that it was fine and even though no scientific evidence is available to support it, she had heard of cases in which folks using herbs have done well. And as a minister, I've read scriptures about how herbs are used to boost the good health of the body. So I decided to prayerfully enter the unknown with the same faith that I approach more tested and approved medical treatments.

I prayed to God the night before going to the Amish practitioner, asking whatever the Master wanted to happen to take place. I developed a more positive mindset and removed my doubts before leaving. To get to his office, I had to take a course alongside winding hills on some of Indiana's seldom-traveled back roads. Leaving the concrete jungle of the city and passing cow pastures and corn stalks put me in another time frame.

When I arrived, the practitioner went over my list of medications. I brought a chronological report detailing my experiences since being diagnosed with prostate cancer. It bothered me that he just glanced over it, but I didn't question it. He didn't really comment, just went on with his examination.

After checking me out, the Amish practitioner urged me not to take the radiation but instead to rely on herbs to accomplish the same goals. I did delay radiation, but eventually underwent the treatment. The Amish practitioner admonished me not to discontinue any of my traditional prescribed drugs as I followed his treatment.

He instructed me to take a half of a cup of chlorophyll daily for a month. Yes, chlorophyll—a green liquid that reminded me of swamp water. It tasted worse than it looked. It was supposed to replace the body strength radiation took away and enhance my immune system. I drank the chlorophyll because I wanted to get well. It made me feel better.

The practitioner suggested I take seven different herbs along with the chlorophyll and a quart of carrot juice every day. His bedside manner and professionalism touched me. He was a no-nonsense individual. There was no charge for the office visits, only for the herbs purchased from the Amish store next door to his office.

Of course, the Amish grow natural, or what we call organic, food. They are very meticulous about their diets and I'm impressed that they have such a tremendous discipline. They don't need some of the things that we couldn't last a day without, like electricity, telephones and cars. They have a strong belief in their faith and they stick to it. You have to admire that.

Another beneficial lifestyle change is to get plenty of exercise. Exercise helps build muscles and contributes to a healthy heart and circulation.

In addition:

- Exercise moves waste products through the intestines more quickly, reducing the time that the intestinal walls are exposed to cancer causing agents
- Exercise promotes insulin efficiency, which decreases the risk of all diseases
- Exercise boosts your immune system by increasing the amount of lymphocytes, interleukin, neutrophils and other immune substances circulating in your body. Big words that accomplish a simple task.
- Building muscle mass burns fat and helps the body maintain leanness, which contributes to good health.
Increased muscle mass enables a higher level of safe fat consumption.

Good nutrition is a must if one is to remain physically and emotionally healthy. Too often we wait until some catastrophic illness attacks our bodies before we acknowledge the need for good diet and healthy eating habits. Too often we compromise the state of our health until we are forced to alter our behavior. It is imperative to develop good, healthy eating habits early in our lives for ourselves as well as for our families. These habits can truly help you and yours live better and healthier over the course of your lives.

Chapter Nine

EPIPHANY

SELF DISCOVERY AND
A NEW PERSPECTIVE

One of the greatest experiences of my life was visiting South Africa in 2001 as guest of Mrs. Judy O'Bannon, the wife of Indiana Governor Frank O'Bannon. A delegation of Indiana leaders examined issues plaguing Africans, including the AIDS epidemic. Just to connect with a country on the "Mother Continent" reinforces one simple reality: The need to maintain our roots.

Two proverbs from the Motherland help me set the tone for my future. The first is from Mali. It says, *"Life is like a ballet performance—danced only once."* The second is Nigerian, warning us that, *"All is never said."*

Often we go through life with such blinding speed and reckless abandon that you would think we had a spare life in the closet or glove compartment, in case this one doesn't work out. But this is it. What we are experiencing is the only life that we'll ever know—at least of this world. We occasionally need to remind ourselves that this is not a dress rehearsal.

If we recognized that fact more often, we wouldn't waste so much time on trivial matters that weigh us down. We would be much more prone to exalt the most important elements of our existence. So many of us don't realize that the dance of life is a short performance. It should be relished.

As to the second proverb, how many of us spend all of our working day trying to get it all done, leaving no "I" undotted; no "T" uncrossed. We seem to think that if we really had enough time, we could do everything that needed to be done. And all too frequently, the result is that our work becomes our life.

A recent national news magazine ran a feature on how Americans are spending more time than ever on the job. Our occupations have become our dominant preoccupation. Hours are piling up at the office, in the factories, on the road or wherever the job site is located. Since there are only twenty-four hours in a day, dedicating a disproportionate amount of time to one area of life automatically lessens the available time for concerns beyond our careers. We work overtime and take on second jobs in a society that places occupation before relations. So the people that we love learn to do without. Significant others and spouses grow accustomed to being alone. Rather than caring parents, all too often babysitters, television, music, video games and the streets are allowed to raise our children.

Leaving the bedside of a business magnate who had just passed away, a hospital chaplain told the nurse as he exited, "You know I've never met a person who in his dying breath lamented that he was sorry there wasn't more time in his life to spend at the office."

America has become a nation of work addicts. I view myself as a recovering workaholic. The result of this is that, sadly, many of us sacrifice our home and family lives.

Work and stress also relate directly to our health. As we become more overwhelmed by the workplace and its stresses, many of us also sacrifice our health. We may give lip service to the thought that nothing is more important than our health. But in terms of how we choose to live, health may not even make the top ten list of things to address over the course of a month. In a society preoccupied with work, there is invariably a price. We make bad choices that can't be undone. I'm a living example.

I was too busy working to attend to my personal health needs, or at least that's what I convinced myself to believe. When you stop to think about it, being too busy to attend to your own health is like being so anxious to get to your destination that you don't bother to put gas in your car. Tired adages urging people to live each day as though it were their last are lost on a society based on the false concept of immortality. Most Americans are so blessed that they take health, happiness and abundance for granted.

Prostate cancer has been an epiphany for me. It's opened my eyes.

As I reexamine my life, it perplexes me. How have I done so well in my professional life and been such a failure in my personal life? I've been married five times. I've never let God lead me in my attempts at marriage the way I submitted to his will in my professional life.

In essence, I'm seeing clearly for the first time. Yes, life is the first and last dance of our ballet. No, we can never do it all or say it all. And in the end, we have to learn to be true to ourselves.

It took prostate cancer to make me realize that, for once, I should put myself first. In saying that, I don't mean it in a self-ish way. I'm just saying that I want to be obedient to God and all of the things He directs me to do. I want to be healed and teach other men how to avert my fate or better cope with life and prostate cancer.

I love Expo to death and the organization is vitally important. Expo has been my life for the past two decades. But the capable people at IBE will have to carry on with a lot less input from me. I'm going to take care of the person inside of me that has been neglected for so long.

This has been a tough transformation for me; a hard realization; but a necessary one. It's important for our health to feel good about ourselves and our environment—to take time out to reflect and smell the roses. Over the past few months, I've had my house remodeled. The carpets are brighter, there is a fresh coat of paint on the walls. I wanted more day-to-day visualization of God's incredible world, so windows were added all around the house to let me enjoy a better view of nature. I spend most of my time on the enclosed back porch appreciating the breathtaking array of sunset hues and the frosty tint of the moon glow against a blackened sky. I can see beauty in the purity of untouched snow on the hill, in the branches of the majestic towering oak trees, in the playfulness of the squirrels scampering up and down their bark, and so many other wonders of the Creator.

My transition has given me the feeling of being in greater contact with God. It's indescribable. The only regret is that it took my somber encounter with prostate cancer to renew my love and appreciation for simple pleasures. But if my example enables others to avoid my mistakes; if it helps them put themselves and their health first, then it will be worth it.

My hope is that sharing my epiphany may provide guideposts for young people on the brink of adulthood, as well as for those who've been around for a while but haven't taken time to open themselves up to life's bounty and beauty.

Grim as the truth may be, no one lives forever. We should stop acting as though we do and fooling ourselves to believe that there's always time later. That's living a lie. And there's nothing like the prospect of your own mortality to force you to put matters into focus. Enriched anticipation of an uncertain future makes you view the present more soulfully. I have a new take on life. I don't get as upset about things as I used to.

Most importantly, I find more time to talk with my son about issues that we probably would have waited to discuss.

You question yourself about how much you should tell a child about a terminal disease without alarming him or her. Well, Charles II was seventeen when I got the bad news. So I just decided to tell him the truth. I wanted him to know the worst-case scenario and what my faith dictated. I wanted him to know the downside of treatments and how they might affect my moods and physical condition, and to know the possibilities such treatments promised.

Through the demands of schoolwork, sports, girls, cars, video games and hip-hop, I wanted Charles II to always have time to reflect.

There is nothing I regret more in life than not spending more time with Charlie. I justified my absence by thinking that I was creating a legacy that would accrue to his benefit. I was establishing the "Williams" name and reputation and making my small contribution to a better world. I reasoned that if my efforts bolstered black Americans, then my son would automatically benefit.

That theory may contain some truth. But it just wasn't enough.

Charles II and I have always had a good relationship. Even before the onset of prostate cancer, we never ended a telephone conversation without saying to each other, "I love you." The problem was that conversation between my son and I was too infrequent, and probably too structured. For both I take responsibility.

Charles II absorbed the news of my illness with his usual stoic expression. Because it is the opposite of my gregarious, 'wear emotions on the sleeve' persona, his 'cool' always left me trying to reach inside of him and pull out more than he was willing to give at a particular moment.

Charles II tended to be more open with his mother. He never seemed to allow raw sentiment to emerge during our one-on-one moments. No matter how often you attempt to dispel the myth, too many men believe that any display of emotion is a sign of weakness. We need to instill in our young men that strength and sensitivity are not mutually exclusive, that the two have a natural mix.

One thing is certain and gratifying. Charles II and I have had more dialogue over the months since my diagnosis than we have had for years. It heartens me to see this young man, who does everything that normal people his age do, get off the telephone, turn off the video game and come to sit down and talk with me. He is always thoughtful to check on my needs as he goes and comes. We never miss a day of telling each other, "I love you."

I want to savor every shared moment. It's important that my youngest son remain humble, and understand that when it rains in your life, God is just trying to grow something; that adversity is only an instrument to make you stronger and fortify your faith.

Our children have to know that they are part of the Master Plan and that something important awaits them in life if they prepare, persevere and give God the praise. I want Charles II to look ahead with confidence, knowing that he never walks alone, but to always look behind him with gratitude for his blessings and for his ancestors who made a better life for him possible.

Conveying life messages to my son is most important to me. Another such message is for him to honor God for his talents and blessings. Finally, I want Charles II to recognize that life is not complete until one recognizes the need to give something back. "To whom much is given, much is required" and the willingness to create and participate in acts of service to others is one of the most vital aspects of the human equation.

Part of the problem we face as a community is that we tend to get so locked into our own agenda that nothing else matters. There's more concern for outdoing a neighbor than helping that neighbor. When we start keeping score of our good deeds in life, everyone loses.

People need to understand that life isn't a game; that winning is meaningless if we hurt others in the process of achieving gain. Too many live the philosophy of the great football coach Vince Lombardi who said "winning isn't everything . . . it's the only thing." And what happens if we offend another en route to our personal conquest? Unfortunately, as we become more of a "me, myself and I" society, "sorry" seems to be the hardest word. Being stricken with cancer has mellowed my approach to life. Things that used to anger me don't get me riled up any more.

Why should it take staring death in the face to make you embrace life?

The obsession with winning, being right or always insisting on having things our way, is a recipe for disaster among people who prefer a more compassionate world where people come first. Too often today reconciliation is a last resort rather than a first priority. And too often our cavalier attitudes lead us to walk away, rather than try to meet someone else half way.

Too often people don't realize this until it's too late. Too many have lost important people in their lives without taking the time to right some wrong or simply to say something that needed to be shared. Some never recover from a missed opportunity.

Sadly, lifelong friends stop speaking over trivial disputes. Family members "fall out" or bicker incessantly. Husbands and wives go to bed angry, then awaken and leave home in the same state. Even some people of God, in congregations throughout the nation and throughout the world, allow petty differences to drive wedges between them and other parishioners.

What if you knew that this week would be your last? Think about it. How would it change your thoughts and actions?

Would you get the same thrill from the 'shop 'til you drop' workout that so captivates our society? Would it shift your sense of values?

Would you still savor the flavor of each meal or allow the sense of doom to overwhelm your sense of taste or perhaps lose your appetite altogether?

Would you awaken brim full of anticipation about the prospects for the day or face tomorrow with a sense of futility?

Would you be quite as anxious to hang out at the local bar or to break a sweat on the nightclub dance floor or prefer more quality time with loved ones?

What would change?

No one really knows because no one knows exactly when he or she will leave this world for eternity. Even if the doctors say that your body is so weak it might not last another season, the truth is that only God has the power to give life or take it away.

But if your sense of physical demise were overwhelming, would it have a significant impact on how you perceive yourself and others each day?

Everyone is different. But hopefully, it would make all of us think more charitably—not just toward those we know but toward nameless others whose suffering is soothed only by the generosity of strangers.

I would like to think that we would be less likely to have negative confrontations, with their lingering effects, and more likely to accent positive relationships with our family members, friends, colleagues, neighbors and strangers.

Perhaps if we saw time as too precious to waste, we would even become more tolerant of petty differences that breed hatred and discrimination.

Perhaps we would learn to recognize the commonalities and celebrate the differences between rich and poor, black and white, men and women, young and old, gay and straight, urban and rural.

If you knew you would never see another daybreak you might look at the sunset with more heart, sing out loud even if you can't carry a tune, laugh out loud over something that would have riled or frustrated you in the past.

You might lift a lasting toast to all those who have gone thankless for the wonderful contributions they made to you over the years; who have no idea how important their simple, heartfelt deeds or expressions were to sustaining you and your dreams. They need to know.

If you knew your life clock was winding down, you might have an urge to call someone you've allowed yourself to grow distant from because of what they did to you or said about you or didn't do for you. You might tell them that—after all of this time —you can forgive them or that you hope they find it in their heart to forgive you.

You'd probably embrace your family members until they pleaded with you to loosen the grip, and even then you might not stop.

Anticipating transition from this world might inspire you to say a prayer that would shake the foundation of Heaven—thanking the Lord for all of the blessings you've received throughout your lifetime as well as for the stumbling blocks He led you around.

You might feel light enough to lift your arms skyward, gaze to the clouds and unleash a "Hallelujah!" or "Thank you, Jesus!" without thought of who sees or hears you.

If any of these are things that you might do if you were certain you had only a few days to live, here's a plan: Do these things today and tomorrow. Don't put them off any longer. The Bible tells us that none of us knows the day or hour of our departure and it's true. So live each day, hour, minute, and second as though it were your last. It may be.

Chapter Ten

LEGACY

THE VIEW FROM WITHIN
AND BEYOND

Even men of science agree. There is a mysterious healing power in our spirit—one that defies the best research of modern medicine.

Think about all the stories of people you knew or heard of who were given a year, a month or less to live. Think of how doctors were stunned by their inexplicable survival.

Think about people who remained in a coma for days, weeks, months even years in some rare cases—then awakened to resume their natural functions.

Men and women of medicine are among the most learned and skilled professionals in society—in this country and around the world. Their training, expertise, and precision leaves us marveling at their proficiency. On a job in which mistakes can literally be a matter of life and death, medical professionals excel. That they care so deeply is a bonus.

But few of these professionals would even venture the notion that they can say with certainty the exact outcome of the best procedures, treatments, or cases diagnosed. Their estimate of a patient's prognosis is a hypothesis based on the information at their disposal. It does not, however, take into account that sometimes God steps in. That's when even professionals are left without an explanation, like the rest of us.

Even leading medical journals acknowledge the unmistakable influence of the mind and spirit in human healing. And those intangibles are influenced by positive thinking, an upbeat attitude, faith in recovery and a solid sense of self.

Self-perception is an important aspect of positive thinking. Part of how you view yourself is contained in how you think others see you. How they assess your deeds and remember you becomes your legacy.

Pondering that legacy, at any point in your life, can be an exercise in self-affirmation. It may be constructive for all of us to look in the mirror occasionally for something other than vanity.

During some of the many interviews since I was diagnosed with prostate cancer, I've had some reporters ask if I think much about dying. My response invariably is that such thoughts dart menacingly in and out of my head almost every hour of every day. I quickly add, however, that they are suppressed with a more significant consideration. That is, how do I view the threat of death in proportion to, and in relation to, the joy of life?

The truth is I've rarely felt so alive!

My joy is born out of the faith that Jesus is not a fair-weather friend. He accompanies us in victory and will not abandon us in struggle. It's hard to convey the comfort of His presence. For those who walk in the light, suffering is redemptive. Even the bad is good.

God led me to write this book in service to more of his children. At the same time, he made it a blessing to me. My nonstop research and writing of *That Black Men Might Live* was actually therapeutic. I am filled with anticipation about the outcome of our labor, about how this book may help galvanize black men to talk among themselves about those things of consequence in their lives, especially about prostate cancer screening and awareness.

Some confuse the word 'living' with 'existence.' A simple houseplant has life. But it can't form a thought or opinion or perform any meaningful action based on it. Too many humans go through life satisfied to make no more contribution to humanity than the average houseplant. They often have their priorities twisted. The real question is not how long a person lives, but how well.

The first thing everyone should do with each sunrise is pause in a prayer of gratitude. Be spiritually thoughtful. If you rose from bed with all your five senses intact, it means God watched over you through the night and decided your journey should continue. If you have to read from your sick bed, you are blessed to have another day among the living. Respect it; use it to better yourself, your family, and mankind.

In the final analysis, the tribulations of my life are all but forgotten. My future is in God's hands and I feel good about it. He has great work for me yet to do. In the glorious present, I see the tremendous value of putting it all in context not only for myself but also for others.

The truth is that every man and woman, famous or not, leaves a legacy because we all benefit from association with many other people. Our parents, neighbors, friends, mentors and teachers all had an impact on us. They may not have been 'stars' but they made a difference in our lives.

To us they were angels. They inspired us, frequently encouraged us, always motivated us, occasionally comforted us, without hesitation instructed us, refused to pompously judge us and even when we fell short, never lost faith or stopped believing in us.

Too often, such individuals leave no lasting document to chronicle their struggle, their contribution . . . their legacy.

Have you even thought about it? When you have left this place and time for the next, what is it that you want people of goodwill to remember? Before I wrote this book, the question was posed to me. It compelled me to consider the legacy I hope to have carved.

It's tough to contemplate your own legacy. The process seems self-indulgent. After all, it forces you into the awkward act of trying to look at yourself through the eyes of others. The very notion of a legacy suggests that you've peaked—that you've reached the height of your possibilities—or that your time is up and you never will. Neither proposition is particularly appealing.

While the awkward emotions of predicting your legacy can't be denied, the reality is that for African Americans in particular, telling our own stories is critical to black America. Journaling our experience sustains whatever contribution we make, offering a road map for those who travel the same road behind us.

It's much too ambitious to think people will remember all the trailblazers—whether celebrities or not. Memory is short. Our lives are so busy that we often forget what we did last week, much less what we did years or even decades ago. It's even harder to recall precisely what someone else did for us.

Since total recall is impossible, the next best thing is documentation. Think of how fascinated "baby boomers" in black America were to discover that, unlike the natives portrayed in the

Tarzan movies, blacks in Africa were kings and queens, scientists, educators, historians and the creators of civilization. Somebody had to tell us the story for us to get the full picture.

That's another reason this book was necessary. It's simply not enough that many perceive Indiana Black Expo as the best black festival in the country every summer and a dynamite football and party weekend every fall.

From those early days of helping to bring entertainment to troops in Nam to organizing the nation's oldest civil rights organization's convention; from helping generate dollars for black scholars to making African Americans more aware of their culture and heritage—service is the cornerstone of any legacy that I might impart.

It's a simple dynamic. Through the grace of God, I found myself in a position to facilitate the dreams of others. In doing so, I fulfilled my own dream.

A classic example is my first encounter with Kenneth "Babyface" Edmonds, arguably the most prolific and successful producer on the modern music scene. When I brought the Jackson Five to Indianapolis the first time, he was in that audience and was awed by the craftsmanship of the singing family from Gary, Indiana.

When he heard the Jacksons were coming again, he couldn't do more than occupy a nosebleed seat high in the balcony. He wanted to meet Michael. Even though he was, at that time, only in the eighth grade, Babyface had already performed with several local groups and knew that he was destined for stardom. He won a local talent show doing the J5 hit, "I Want You Back."

So Babyface came up with a scheme. He found my name in a newspaper article as the promoter of a Jackson Five concert in his home town of Indianapolis. 'Face' called me, dropping his youthful voice a few octaves—pretending to be his teacher. Calling himself Mr. Clayton, he explained that there was this exceptional student named Kenneth Edmonds who wanted to meet Michael Jackson.

Instinctively, I responded, saying that I would do whatever I could to help. Kenneth "Babyface" Edmonds tells the rest of the story:

When Rev. Williams called me to say that my teacher told him about me, I acted surprised. I had to make sure that I spoke in my voice and not 'Mr. Clayton's' It was one of those unbelievable things. He made my dream come true. Charles arranged for me to meet Michael and his talented bothers. It's impossible to convey how much that brief encounter influenced my career as an entertainer, but it had a great impact.

That's typical of what Rev. Williams has done since I've known him. He was always looking out for someone else. For a while, he promoted my singing group. We maintained a close friendship over the years and then one day he called to tell me that he and Indiana State Representative Bill Crawford, who was Chairman of the Board of Indiana Black Expo, were trying to change Interstate 65 to Kenneth "Babyface" Edmonds Highway. Rev. Williams had the vision and Representative Crawford assisted him in his efforts to make it a reality. Hard as it was for me to believe, they did it. I was proud. My mother was even prouder.

When I heard that Rev. Williams had prostate cancer and was putting together public service announcements, helping to organize screening clinics for other black men and writing a book, I was devastated at the news of his cancer, but his response to it didn't surprise me at all. It's typical for Charles to encourage and uplift others, even in the midst of his own misfortune.

We tell our stories not for our own edification, not for glory, but for our children. To know themselves, they need to know their ancestors and their heritage. They need to hear the voices of the generations that came before them. It is for this reason that I tell my story.

I hope that people of goodwill recall that I tried to help people, that I uplifted our heritage and that I remained humble. I hope that those kind enough to flip through the pages of my life story will say about me:

- *"He tried to help somebody as he passed along."*
  Inspired by Dr. King from the beginning, there's nothing greater anyone can say about me than I tried to help somebody. I tried to be a friend to all and gave from my heart without expectation, acknowledging the message of Christ that tells us, "That which you have done unto the least of mine, so have you done unto me."
- *"He revered the past, embraced the future, but lived in the present."*
  I tried to create vehicles to help us recognize and honor our black icons and pacesetters. On the other end, I touted education as key to unlocking portals to the future—reflecting scripture that urges self-sufficiency in saying, 'Give a man a fish and you feed him for a day . . . teach him how to fish and you feed him for a lifetime.'
- *"He never forgot where he came from."*
  Some who reach a modicum of success—by one yard-

stick or another—disavow their link to people, places and things that lifted them up. Borrowing the prose of Rudyard Kipling, I hope people will say that 'all men matter to me but none too much—that I've been blessed to walk with kings but I've never lost the common touch.'

One of the things that pleases me most is that my life has been centered on coalition-building. It's never been important to me that I be praised individually. It's infinitely more important that Expo is acknowledged. However humbling, I point to the Lord whenever someone does applaud my capacity to pull together dissimilar parts into a collective effort toward a common cause.

My legacy and that of IBE are intertwined.

The organization has been my life. Even as I take time to go inward more during this period of my life, I hope people will know that I gave all that I had to give during every waking hour. I can only make a lasting impression when IBE has made sustaining contributions to the betterment of black Americans.

The measure of IBE's contributions must extend beyond the intellectual stimulation of seminars and workshops, the entertainment of concerts and stage shows, the cultural exhibition featuring visual arts indigenous to black people, and the economic boosts provided by the sprawling marketplace IBE events offer to the African American entrepreneur.

That legacy must also include the role Expo played in enabling aspiring black scholars to receive funding for their educational pursuits; IBE's efforts to feed the hungry and clothe those in need. Expo has pushed for African Americans to return to basics by reclaiming our youth, strengthening the institution of the black family and insisting that God steers our course in both.

No single element of the IBE legacy or future carries more significance than the annual Health Fair. The cooperation of health care professionals throughout central Indiana is awesome. So is the enthusiasm of organizations and individuals that volunteer to make the Health Fair run smoothly. And the response from the thousands of participants bodes well for increased health consciousness among black Americans.

African Americans seem to be moving closer to the realization that religion, education, economics, culture, entertainment, social issues, government and other concerns rely on the health of those assuming the mantle of responsibility in each area. If IBE plays a role in this process of enlightenment, then that constitutes a legacy in which we can all take pride.

Some people look at life tests as a form of punishment. Adversity can rock the very spiritual foundation of some of the most devout Christians—especially when one's physical health is attacked. All of us, from time to time, have wondered when some pain we felt would finally subside. It's only human.

But all it takes to get a clear perspective of how God works is to examine the stories of some of the most tested people of faith. The three Hebrew boys placed into the fiery furnace must, at some point, have prepared for their doom without knowing that when that place was revisited, the punishing king would find them unburned and with a fourth companion. God Almighty.

Following the inexplicable word of God, Abraham was perplexed even in obedience as he prepared his son as a sacrifice. No matter how heavy each step, he went to the designated place, laid his son as an offering and raised the knife that would have meant the boy's death before the Lord held back his hand and commended his faith.

Mary and Martha wept and even mourned in disbelief after Jesus came to the burial place of their brother. Rather than having wholehearted belief and confidence in the Lord, they lamented the fact that their brother would still be alive had Christ arrived earlier. Through their weeping they watched as Lazarus' name was called three times. Then they watched in awe as he rose from his deathbed and walked like a natural man.

All of us have moments of feeling forsaken. Don't let them last. My comfort comes in knowing that God said weeping may endure for a night but joy will come in the morning. Prostate cancer makes my days long and my nights longer. It's not easy having something in your life so compelling that it drives almost every thought and every emotion. Yet, through it all, I am able to remain calm, knowing that God is beside me as he was beside the Hebrew boys.

Like Abraham, shaky as it may be sometime, mine is a walk of faith. Just as he approached that chilling altar with trepidation but kept coming, I enter each day with a certain amount of fear but keep faith that the Lord will also reveal to me a ram in the bush—some saving grace.

And as it was proven to Mary and Martha that there is nothing too hard for God, so do I expect to rise from the clutches of dreary fate and rise to do the work of God.

Through every test, I will give praise. Through every tear, I will give praise. Through every triumph, I will praise Him. In every setback, his name will remain on the tip of my lips. A lyric of a traditional gospel song says it in the words, *"Lord, don't move that mountain . . . give me strength to climb it. Please don't move that stumbling block . . . just lead me on around it."*

With all I am going through, if you accept nothing else, believe this. God is going to work it out. For kindred spirits, no proof of the realness of faith is necessary. For cynics, no proof will ever be acceptable. So I choose to continue in my path of service as long as God allows. And if my legacy really means anything, hopefully it will encourage everyone to live until it's time for every person's individual transition.

Whenever the time comes, all will be well if you are able to say that you did what you could when you could. Be able to say that you made mistakes, but that you repented. Be able to say that you tried to live helping others. And be able to say that you put God first.

In the waning years, your rewards won't need to come in the form of plaques, trophies or certificates. Platitudes in the form of highly placed testimonials, inclusion in history books and tributes from dignitaries have their place. But they don't paint the entire picture. Neither praise from everyday people nor towering statues, monuments or shrines bearing your name make the difference, because only what you do for Christ will last.

There is no greater legacy for Christians than to live in such a way that when they reach their journey's end—at whatever point our Lord and Savior chooses—they can stand before the throne on that momentous day in glory and hear the simple, two-word phrase: "Well done."

JOURNAL SAMPLE

"My Personal Journal of the Journey"

Starting and maintaining a journal of my treatment since my diagnosis has been a very helpful and valuable tool. It provides a continuous record of both the medication that has been prescribed as well as the course of treatment. I encourage those of you who have been diagnosed with prostate cancer to keep such a record. What follows is simply a sample of my journal. I hope it gives you an idea of how you can track the information that is important to you.

The form of the journal doesn't really matter. Use one that best suits your needs. The key is to keep one. Valerie prefers keeping my records on a computer. This method provides easy access and legibility. Also if a doctor or family member has questions or concerns, and requests the information, Valerie can quickly e-mail it.

"My Personal Journal of the Journey"

Date	Reason for Visit	Assessment
May 28, 2002	Cat Scan taken at St. Vincent Hospital Lab Test	
May 30, 2002	Advised of Cat Scan and PSA results by Dr. Thomas Petrin PSA—175	Diagnosis: Prostatic Carcinoma with metastic disease involving the ribs and the lymph nodes Referred to Dr. Andrew Moore (Urologist)
June 10, 2002	Biopsy performed by Dr. Andrew Moore at Methodist Hospital	
June 13, 2002	Referred to Dr. Frank Lloyd J.	Need to have fluid drawn from my lymph nodes for evaluation.